*M*artinis before lunch?
Brandy after dinner?
Thick, juicy steak, sauce bearnaise,
salad with any kind of dressing?

It's amazing! It's delightful! It works!
This is the diet you've been waiting for.
Forget about calories. All you need to
watch (besides the scale) on this
extraordinary new diet is your intake of
carbohydrates. You eat as much protein
and fat as you please, while just 60 grams
a day keeps the pounds away—and you
can lose up to five pounds a week.

THE NEW CARBOHYDRATE GRAM COUNTER
is the book with all the answers for anyone
who hates dieting. An uncomplicated,
easy-to-follow guide that will hearten
and lighten weight-watchers everywhere.

THE NEW CARBOHYDRATE GRAM COUNTER

A DELL BOOK AN ORIGINAL VOLUME

Published by DELL PUBLISHING CO., INC.
1 Dag Hammarskjold Plaza, New York, N.Y. 10017
Copyright © 1965, by Dell Publishing Co., Inc.
Dell ® TM 681510, Dell Publishing Co., Inc.
First Dell Printing—June, 1965
Second Dell Printing—December, 1965
Third Dell Printing—May, 1967
Fourth Dell Printing—December, 1967
Fifth Dell Printing—September, 1968
Sixth Dell Printing—April, 1969
Seventh Dell Printing—August, 1969
Eighth Dell Printing—March, 1970
Ninth Dell Printing—July, 1970
Tenth Dell Printing—February, 1971
Eleventh Dell Printing—July, 1971
Twelfth Dell Printing—October, 1971
Thirteenth Dell Printing—January, 1972
Fourteenth Dell Printing—June, 1972
Fifteenth Dell Printing—August, 1972
Sixteenth Dell Printing—October, 1972
Seventeenth Dell Printing—January, 1973
Eighteenth Dell Printing—April, 1973

Printed in the U.S.A.

CONTENTS

THE DIET FOR PEOPLE WHO HATE TO DIET   9

GRAM COUNTS FROM A TO Z   17

ALCOHOLIC BEVERAGES   101

LOW-GRAM SNACKS & TIDBITS   104

TWO WEEKS OF LOW-GRAM MENUS   107

TOTAL YOUR GRAMS   124

WHAT YOU SHOULD WEIGH   127

THE NEW CARBOHYDRATE GRAM COUNTER

THE DIET FOR PEOPLE WHO HATE TO DIET

Like millions of men and women, are you overweight, but unable to face the prospect of the usual dreary diet: celery stalks, carrot strips and cucumber slices; skim milk, black coffee and sauerkraut juice? Yes? Then the new low-carbohydrate diet is designed especially for you—for people who despise dieting, who find salad without dressing unbearable, eggs without bacon unthinkable, dinner without a martini uncivilized.

The amazing low-carbohydrate diet is not like any diet you've tried in the past. Rumored to have originated at the United States Air Force Academy, this diet permits you to eat as much protein and fat as you please. All you need to watch is your intake of carbohydrates—sugars and starches. Forget about calories; they have no part in this diet. What you count are carbohydrate grams; what you do is limit your starch and sugar intake to 60 grams daily. It's as simple as that—and, as you'll see, almost as pleasant as not dieting at all! Mayonnaise and hollandaise, sour cream and heavy cream, a thick slice of ham, a rich leg of lamb—these and dozens of other usually "forbidden" foods are yours on a low-carbohydrate diet.

How can such a delightful diet work? In simplified form, here is the explanation. The energy your body needs to function is supplied largely by carbohydrates and fats (the main function of proteins is to rebuild tissue). Recent studies indicate that excessive consumption of carbohydrates is the primary cause of overweight. In other words, when your body doesn't burn up all the starches and sugars you eat, the excess carbohydrates turn quickly into unwelcome pounds. On a low-carbohydrate diet, your body is forced to call upon its own fat—stored-up carbohydrates—for energy; thus, you lose weight. A second reason for the success of a low-carbohydrate diet is that proteins and fat "stick to the ribs" (in actuality, remain in the stomach) longer than sugars and starches; therefore, you're not perpetually hungry. Some scientists argue that a low-carbohydrate diet results in an intake of fewer calories, which in turn results in a loss of weight. Unquestionably, many low-carbohydrate dieters cut down on calories by drastically limiting their consumption of foods such as cake, candy, bread, potatoes, etc. However, there are cases on record of dieters who have shed pounds while enjoying high-calorie, low-carbohydrate meals. Science still has much to learn about body chemistry and food, but this much at least is certain: calories alone do not account for weight loss or gain. Nutritionists and other scientists may not always agree about why a low-carbohydrate diet works, but there is general agreement that it does work!

What can you eat on a low-carbohydrate diet? Unlimited amounts of every kind of meat, poultry, fish or seafood; unlimited amounts of pure fats and oils; eggs; most cheeses; many vegetables. Like your steak broiled with a wedge of butter? Go ahead—enjoy it and still diet. Like your pork chops and chicken fried, your celery stuffed with Roquefort cheese? Enjoy them all—and while you're at it, have a martini, a Manhattan, a highball. The principle of low-carbohydrate dieting is truly very simple: You may eat pure proteins and fats to your heart's content; partake of hundreds of foods that contain little or no starch and/or sugar.

What can't you eat on a low-carbohydrate diet? In general, try to forget cereals, bread, cakes—most grain products (including, of course, all forms of pasta). Also on your not-to-be-eaten-often list: candy, most fresh and all dried fruits, fruit juices, ice cream and sherbet, pastry, carbonated soft drinks (except for those produced without sugar), beer and ale, starchy vegetables such as corn, potatoes, lima beans and peas.

Counting carbohydrate grams is different from—and easier than—counting calories. Yes, you must keep track of every gram, but so many foods contain no grams, you don't have to be an Einstein to keep tabs on your carbohydrate intake. If you're an experienced hand at dieting, begin now to unlearn some old ideas and habits. For example? For example, a cup of skim milk contains one more carbohydrate gram than a cup of whole milk—and four more grams than heavy cream! In other words, on a low-carbohydrate diet, it's better to add cream to your coffee than whole milk; better to add whole milk than skim milk! Other examples: carrots are too "expensive" for nibbling (each contains five grams), but cheddar cheese isn't (half a gram per ounce); an old diet standby, chilled fruit gelatin, contains a whopping 36 grams per cup, but a tablespoon of peanut butter atop a saltine totals just six grams. Remember, calories don't necessarily count on a low-carbohydrate diet; therefore, experienced dieters must beware of foods that are low in calories, but relatively high in carbohydrate grams—for instance, raw onions (11 grams each), canned sauerkraut (7 grams a cup) beets (5 grams each), dill pickles (3 grams each).

The magic number on a low-carbohydrate diet is 60—cut your carbohydrate intake to 60 grams daily and you should lose 10-15 pounds a month. According to the "Yearbook of Agriculture" (a publication of the United States Department of Agriculture), "People and animals very likely can survive quite well on diets containing no carbohydrates, because the body can also use fats and proteins directly as sources of energy . . ." Thus, to shed weight more quickly, you can cut your carbohydrate intake still further—but, to play safe, nutritionists recommend that you consume no less than 30 carbohydrate grams a day. Like many diets, a low-carbohydrate diet may seem to lose its effectiveness after two or three weeks. If that is how it works with you—if your weight stays at the same level for a few days, even for a week —don't become discouraged; don't give up. Soon, you'll begin to lose again (and, in most cases) at the earlier speedy rate.

Before starting this diet (or any diet) get your doctor's approval. And after you've begun, use your good sense in choosing the foods you eat. Protect your heart by watching your intake of saturated fats (dieting or not dieting, you should do that); protect your liver by including many protein-rich foods (eggs, cheese, fish and meat); protect your over-all health by including foods rich in vitamins and minerals, by supplementing your diet with a multivitamin every day. Finally, bear in mind that if you remain on a low-carbohydrate diet more than two weeks, you should be sure to include limited—but daily— quantities of milk and citrus fruit.

Satisfy your sweet tooth on a low-carbohydrate diet by utilizing artificial sweeteners, by sampling sugar-free canned fruits and other desserts, by cultivating a taste for fresh strawberries, cherries, raspberries and canta- loupe—the fruits "cheapest" in carbohydrate content. (When you yearn for a gooey hot fudge sundae, tell your- self that a low-carbohydrate diet not only takes off pounds, but helps reduce tooth decay as well. It's true —ask your dentist.) Learn to snack on little chunks of cheese, on bacon bits, sardines, shrimp, chicken livers, and other high-protein foods. You don't ever have to be hungry on a low-carbohydrate diet; the trick is simply in knowing which foods to eat.

The gram counts in this book were, whenever possible, obtained from handbooks and yearbooks published by the United States Department of Agriculture. However, as you count your grams, bear in mind that no two onions, potatoes, etc., are exactly the same size; there- fore, to be accurate, be honest. If you eat a huge tomato, you're cheating only yourself if you count it as 6 grams (the "price" of a medium-size tomato). As you count, bear in mind these factors, too: in this book, "a cup" means 8 ounces; a teaspoon or tablespoon means a level —not a heaping—teaspoon or tablespoon.

Use this book as you would use a dictionary—looking up all foods alphabetically. Carry your gram counter wherever you go, refer to it before you plan each of your meals; before you reach for any snack. Remember, until you learn the important gram counts by heart, one "little" error—for example a 54-gram wedge of mince pie—can destroy your entire day!

GRAM COUNTS
FROM A TO Z

Listed alphabetically, the carbohydrate content of 1500 foods, plus separate lists of alcoholic drinks (page 101), snacks and tidbits (page 104).

	grams
Abalone, broiled (3½ ounces)	3.0
Abalone, canned (⅔ cup)	2.9
Alcoholic beverages (see separate listing, page 101)	
Almonds	
In shell (1 cup)	7.8
Shelled (½ cup)	14.0
Salted (12 to 15)	2.9
Salted, chopped (1 tablespoon)	1.8
Chocolate covered (10 medium)	16.9
Ambrosia (½ cup)	23.2
Anchovies, canned (8 small fillets)	trace
Anchovy paste (1 teaspoon)	.3
Apple brown betty (see Puddings)	
Apple butter (1 tablespoon)	8.5
Apple cider (see Cider)	
Apple dumpling (see Puddings)	
Apple juice (see Juices)	
Apple pie (see Pies)	
Apples	
Raw (1 large)	27.3

Raw (1 medium) 16.9
Raw (1 small) 11.1
Raw (1 cup slices) 19.0
Baked, 2 tablespoons sugar (1 large) 51.3
Dehydrated (1 pound) 413.0
Dried (1 pound) 332.0
Dried, cooked, unsweetened (1 cup) 50.8
Dried, cooked, sweetened (1 cup) 77.0
Frozen, sweetened (½ cup slices) 25.0
Apples and apricots, canned, strained (1 ounce) 5.0
Applesauce, canned, unsweetened (1 cup) 26.2
Applesauce, canned, sweetened (1 cup) 50.0
Applesauce, canned, strained (1 ounce) 5.5
Apricot nectar (see Juices)
Apricot pie (see Pies)
Apricots
Fresh (3 medium) 13.0
Candied (1 medium) 26.0
Canned (1 cup with syrup) 54.8
Canned (4 halves, 2 tablespoons syrup) 26.4
Canned, water pack (1 cup with liquid) 19.8
Canned, low calorie (½ cup) 9.2
Canned, strained (1 ounce) 9.8
Dried (5 small halves) 12.5
Dried (1 cup, 35 to 40 small halves) 100.0
Dried, cooked, unsweet. (½ cup, with liquid) ..31.1
Dried, cooked, sweetened (½ cup, with liquid) ..51.4

Frozen, sweetened (½ cup) 32.5
Arrowroot (1 tablespoon) 7.0
Artichoke hearts, canned (5) 8.0
Artichokes, French (1) 14.2
Artichokes, Jerusalem (4 small) 16.5
Artichokes, bottom (1) 5.0
Asparagus (6 stalks cooked) 3.0
Asparagus (1 cup cut spears) 6.0
Asparagus, canned (1 cup cut spears) 6.0
Asparagus, canned (6 spears) 3.4
Asparagus, frozen (6 spears) 3.9
Asparagus soup (see Soups)
Avocado, California (½ medium) 6.0
Avocado, California (1 cup cubes) 9.0
Avocado, Florida (½ medium) 11.0
Avocado, Florida (1 cup cubes) 13.0

B

grams
Bacon, broiled or fried (1 pound) 4.8
Bacon, broiled or fried (2 strips) 2
Bacon, Canadian, cooked (1 slice) .... trace

Bacon fat (see Fats)

Bagel (1 medium) 32.5

Baked beans (see Beans)

Bamboo shoots (1 cup) 7.9

Banana fritter (1) 11.4

Banana custard or whip (see Puddings)

Bananas

    Fresh (1 large) 44.4

    Fresh (1 medium) 34.5

    Fresh (1 small) 23.0

    Fresh (1 cup slices) 35.4

    Fried in butter (1 medium) 34.6

Barley, dry (1 cup) 160.0

Bass, baked 0

Bass, broiled 0

Bass, canned 0

Bavarian cream (see Puddings)

Bean curd (1 portion) 2.4

Bean soup (see Soups)

Bean sprouts, mung, cooked (1 cup, drained) 5.2

Bean sprouts, soy, cooked (1 cup, drained) 3.7

Beans

    Baked, canned, pork and molasses (1 cup) 54.0

    Baked, canned, pork and tomato sauce (1 cup) .43.1

    Baked, canned, without pork (1 cup) 52.2

    Green (1 cup cooked) 6.0

    Green, canned (1 cup, with liquid) 9.6

Green, canned, strained (1 ounce) 1.1
Green, frozen, cut (1 cup) 14.1
Green, frozen, French-style (1 cup) 14.4
Kidney (1 cup cooked) 42.0
Lima (1 cup cooked) 29.2
Lima, canned (1 cup) 29.4
Lima, dry (1 cup cooked) 48.0
Lima, frozen (3½ ounces) 17.6
Navy, dry (½ cup) 61.6
Pinto, dry (½ cup) 63.7
Red Mexican, dry (½ cup) 63.7
Soy, dry (½ cup) 36.6
Wax (1 cup cooked) 6.0
Wax, canned (1 cup, with liquid) 9.6
Wax, frozen, cut (1 cup) 14.8
White marrow, dry (½ cup) 61.6

Beef

Boiled 0
Brains (see Brains)
Braised or pot-roasted 0
Brisket 0
Chuck 0
Corned 0
Corned, hash (see Hash)
Dried, chipped 0
Dried, chipped, creamed (½ cup) 6.1
Flank 0

Hamburger 0
Heart (see Heart)
Kidneys (see Kidneys)
Liver (see Liver)
Plate 0
Pot pie, frozen (8 oz.) 40.8
Potted 0
Roast 0
Round 0
Rump 0
Short ribs 0
Steak 0
Stewing 0
Tongue, boiled (3 ounces) 4
Tongue, potted, deviled (1 tablespoon) 1
Beef hash (see Hash)
Beef suet 0
Beef and vegetable stew (see Stew)
Beer (see separate listing, page 101)
Beet greens (1 cup cooked) 5.6
Beets
Raw (2) 9.6
Cooked (1 cup) 16.2
Canned (1 cup, with liquid) 17.9
Canned, strained (1 ounce) 2.4
Pickled (1 cup) 20.0
Bell pepper (see Peppers, green)

Beverages (see individual listings)

Beverages, alcoholic (see separate listing, page 101)

Biscuits, baking powder (1 medium) 19.8

Biscuits, baking powder (1 small) 14.0

Blackberries

    Fresh (1 cup) 18.0

    Canned (1 cup with syrup) 45.6

    Canned, water pack (1 cup with liquid) 22.5

    Canned, low calorie (1 cup) 18.4

Blackberry jelly (see Jams, jellies)

Blackberry pie (see Pies)

Black-eyed peas (see Cowpeas)

Blancmange (see Puddings)

Blintzes (1 small) 12.9

Blueberries

    Fresh (1 cup) 21.1

    Canned (1 cup with syrup) 60.0

    Canned, water pack (1 cup with liquid) 21.8

    Canned, low calorie (1 cup) 17.4

    Frozen, sweetened (1 cup) 37.2

    Frozen, unsweetened (3 ounces) 22.0

Blueberry pie (see Pies)

Bluefish, broiled or baked 0

Bluefish, fried in 1 tbs. butter 1

Bologna, all meat (8 ounces, about 8 slices) 2.0

Bologna, all meat (⅛-inch slice) 2

Bouillon (see Soups)

Bouillon cube, beef or chicken (1 cube) 0
Bourbon (see separate listing, page 102)
Boysenberries, frozen, sweetened (1 cup) 35.2
Boysenberries, frozen, unsweetened (1 cup) 11.8
Brains, all kinds (3 ounces) 7
Bran flakes (see Cereals)
Brandy (see separate listing, page 102)
Brazil nuts (1 medium) 4
Brazil nuts, in shell (10) 4.8
Brazil nuts, shelled (½ cup) 7.5
Bread crumbs, dry (1 cup) 63.8
Bread crumbs, dry (1 tablespoon) 4.0
Bread pudding (see Puddings)
Bread stuffing (see Stuffing)
Breads
    Banana tea (1 slice) 21.8
    Boston brown (¾-inch slice) 21.4
    Bran (1 slice) 17.0
    Bran raisin (1 slice) 27.2
    Brown nut (1 slice) 27.2
    Cinnamon (1 slice) 15.9
    Corn (1 piece) 21.1
    Corn, Southern-style (2-inch square) 21.6
    Cracked wheat (1 slice) 11.8
    Date nut (1 slice) 28.0
    French (1 pound) 236.1
    French (1 small slice) 10.4

Ginger (see Cakes)

Gluten (1 slice) 8.7

Graham (1 pound) 220.0

Graham (1 slice) 11.0

Italian (1 pound) 243.8

Italian (1 small slice) 10.7

Melba toast (see Toast)

Protein (1 slice) 8.7

Pumpernickel (1 pound) 237.9

Pumpernickel (1 slice) 15.9

Raisin (1 pound) 266.0

Raisin (1 slice) 13.3

Roman meal (1 slice) 13.7

Rye, light (1 pound) 237.9

Rye, light (1 slice) 12.1

Rye, dark (1 slice) 15.9

Rye, party sliced (1 slice) 7.9

Rye and wheat (1 slice) 12.1

Short (1 piece) 21.6

Spoon (1 serving) 17.0

Vienna (1 pound) 236.1

Vienna (1 small slice) 10.4

White (1 pound) 235.2

White (1 slice) 11.9

Whole wheat (1 pound) 222.5

Whole wheat (1 slice) 11.3

Whole wheat, raisin (1 slice) 15.0

Zwieback (see Toast)

Breakfast foods (see Cereals)

Broccoli (1 stalk) 5.5

Broccoli (1 cup cooked) 8.2

Broccoli, frozen (2-3 spears) 4.3

Broccoli, frozen, chopped (½ cup) 4.6

Brown betty (see Puddings)

Brown sugar (see Sugar)

Brownies (see Cookies)

Brussels sprouts (1 cup cooked) 12.4

Brussels sprouts, frozen (1 cup) 16.6

Buckwheat flour (see Flour)

Buckwheat pancakes (see Pancakes)

Buffalo meat 0

Buns

    Cinnamon (1) 25.6

    Cinnamon raisin (1) 28.6

    Hot cross (1) 20.0

    Pecan (1) 37.0

Butter (1 cup) 1.8

Butter (1 tablespoon) 1

Butter, sweet (1 tablespoon) 1

Butterfish, baked or broiled 0

Buttermilk (see Milk)

Butternuts (4 or 5) 1.3

Butterscotch candy (see Candies)

Butterscotch sauce (see Sauces)

C

	grams
Cabbage (1 cup shredded)	5.4
Cabbage (1 cup cooked)	9.0
Cabbage, Chinese (1 cup)	2.4
Cabbage, Chinese (1 cup cooked)	4.6
Cabbage, cole slaw (see Salads)	
Cakes	

Almond coffee (1 slice) 32.8
Angel food (1 slice) 33.0
Apple crumb (1 slice) 49.1
Applesauce (1 piece) 18.7
Butter, plain (1 square) 36.3
Butter, iced (1 square) 46.1
Caramel, iced (1 slice) 44.1
Cheesecake (1 piece) 27.8
Cheesecake, pineapple (1 piece) 37.0
Chocolate, plain (1 piece) 22.8
Chocolate, iced (1 piece) 45.0
Chocolate layer cake (1 piece) 54.8
Coconut, iced (1 piece) 50.0
Coffee, plain (1 piece) 31.6

Coffee, iced, with nuts (1 piece) 32.8
Cup, plain (1) 22.8
Cup, iced (1) 31.0
Date torte (1 serving) 38.1
Fruit (1 slice) 22.4
Gingerbread (1 square) 26.9
Gold (1 slice) 14.8
Jelly roll (1 slice) 38.8
Layer, 2 layers (1 piece) 54.4
Layer, 3 layers (1 piece) 72.5
Marble (1 slice) 31.0
Pineapple upside-down (1 piece) 71.2
Pound (1 slice) 14.8
Shortcake (see Shortcake)
Sponge (1 piece) 21.8
Sunshine (1 piece) 36.3
Washington cream (1 piece) 39.1
Calves' liver (see Liver)
Candied apricots (see Apricots)
Candied cherries (see Cherries)
Candied citron (1 ounce) 22.7
Candied ginger (see Ginger root)
Candied peel (1 ounce) 22.9
Candies
Almond Joy (10c size) 33.0
Bon bon (1) 9.4
Brown sugar fudge (1 piece) 22.9

Butterscotch (1 ounce) 24.3
Butterscotch (1 piece) 4.3
Caramel (1 ounce) 22.0
Caramel (1 medium) 7.8
Caramel, chocolate nut (1 piece) 8.8
Chocolate, bitter (1-ounce square) 8.3
Chocolate, bitter, grated (1 cup) 41.5
Chocolate, milk (1 ounce) 15.9
Chocolate, milk, with almonds (1 ounce) 16.9
Chocolate, semisweet (1 ounce) 17.5
Chocolate, sweet (1-ounce square) 17.8
Chocolate almonds (1 ounce) 16.9
Chocolate bar (2-ounce bar) 32.4
Chocolate bar, with nuts (1 ounce) 16.9
Chocolate cherry (1) 8.6
Chocolate cream (1 ounce) 20.0
Chocolate cream (1 medium) 8.6
Chocolate-covered almonds (6) 8.5
Chocolate fudge (1 piece) 23.7
Chocolate kisses (1) 2.2
Chocolate mint (5c size) 23.0
Chocolate mint (3 small) 21.6
Clark bar (5c bar) 21.6
Coconut cream (1 square) 20.0
Cream mint (2 small) 2.7
Date cream (1 ounce) 20.0
Divinity (1 piece) 22.9

Fondant (1 patty) 10.0
Fruit drops (3) 9.9
Fudge (1 piece) 22.9
Fudge, with nuts (1 ounce) 17.5
Glazed fruit (1 large piece) 8.1
Gum drops (1 large or 8 small) 8.6
Hard (1 ounce) 28.0
Hershey milk chocolate (5c bar) 15.9
Hershey milk chocolate, almonds (5c bar) 15.7
Jelly beans (10) 16.5
Lemon drops (1) 5.0
Lifesavers, fruit (1 roll) 35.0
Lifesavers, mint (1 roll) 30.0
Lollipop (1 large) 56.0
Lollipop (1 medium) 28.0
Maple sugar (see Sugar)
Mars bar (1⅛-ounce bar) 21.8
Mars Milky Way (1 bar) 58.3
Mars Three Musketeers (1⅜ ounce) 35.1
Marshmallow (1 ounce) 23.0
Marshmallow (1) 6.2
Marshmallow, chocolate (1) 8.5
Mints, after dinner (5 small) 1.3
Mints, chocolate (see Candies, chocolate mint)
Molasses kisses (1) 6.0
Mounds (10c bar) 29.7
Nestle's milk chocolate (5c bar) 15.4

Nestle's milk chocolate, almonds (5c bar) 15.2
Nestle's milk chocolate, crunch (5c bar) 15.0
Nestle's semisweet bits (1 ounce) 16.8
Oh Henry (1 bar) 21.8
Orange drops (1) 4.9
Packaged (2 rolls) 9.9
Peanut bar (2 ounces) 17.2
Peanut brittle (1 piece) 20.6
Penny (2 ounces) 28.0
Snickers (1 bar) 25.1
Sourballs (1) 9.9
Cantaloupe (½ melon) 8.3
Cantaloupe (1 cup diced) 11.0
Capers (1 tablespoon) ....trace
Caramel (see Candies)
Caramel sauce (see Sauces)
Carbonated soft drinks (see Soft drinks)
Carrot juice (see Juices)
Carrots
Raw (1) 5.1
Raw, grated (1 cup) 10.2
Raw, sticks (3) 2.8
Cooked (1 cup diced) 9.4
Canned (1 cup diced) 9.6
Canned, strained (1 ounce) 1.6
Frozen (½ cup) 4.6
Casaba melon (1 wedge) 12.8

Cashew nuts (1 cup roasted) 35.0
Cashew nuts (1 ounce) 8.3
Cashew nuts (6 to 8) 4.1
Cassava (3½ ounces) 83.5
Catfish 0
Catsup (1 tablespoon) 4.2
Cauliflower (1 cup buds) 4.9
Cauliflower (1 cup cooked) 6.0
Cauliflower, frozen (1 cup) 7.6
Caviar (1 ounce) 1.1
Celeriac (4 to 6 roots) 8.8
Celery (1 large stalk) 1.5
Celery (1 cup diced) 3.7
Celery, cooked (1 cup) 4.8
Cereals
    Bran (¾ cup) 31.4
    Bran flakes (¾ cup) 22.6
    Cerevim, dry (½ cup) 15.3
    Cheerios (1 cup) 17.7
    Corn, puffed (¾ cup) 25.0
    Corn flakes (1 cup) 21.0
    Corn flakes, sugar frosted (1 cup) 35.0
    Corn grits (1 cup) 26.6
    Cream of Wheat, cooked (1 cup) 26.8
    Farina, cooked (1 cup) 29.6
    Grape Nuts (¼ cup) 24.0
    Grape Nuts Flakes (¾ cup) 23.0

Hominy (1 cup) 26.6

Infant's dry, precooked (1 ounce) 20.4

Kellogg's Concentrate (½ cup) 7.0

Kellogg's Special "K" (1 cup) 12.5

Kix (¾ cup) 15.0

Krispies (¾ cup) 25.1

Krumbles (¾ cup) 23.8

Maltex, cooked (¾ cup) 24.0

Mapo oat, cooked (¾ cup) 21.0

Muffets (1) 18.2

Oat, ready to eat (1 cup) 17.5

Oat, rolled (⅔ cup) 17.3

Oatmeal, cooked (1 cup) 26.0

Pablum (2 tablespoons) 4.3

Pep (1 cup) 23.0

Post Toasties (¾ cup) 15.0

Raisin bran (1 cup) 33.2

Ralston, cooked (⅔ cup) 20.1

Ralston Wheat Chex (¾ cup) 35.0

Rice, puffed (1 cup) 11.7

Rice flakes (¾ cup) 21.2

Rice Krispies (1 cup) 25.1

Rolled oats, cooked (⅓ cup) 19.3

Shredded wheat (1-ounce biscuit) 18.3

Sugar Krisps (1 cup) 26.1

Wheat, puffed (1 cup) 9.6

Wheat, puffed, sweetened (1 ounce) 17.6

Wheat, rolled, cooked (½ cup) 20.0
Wheat and malted barley, cooked (¾ cup) 21.7
Wheat flakes (1 cup) 23.0
Wheatena, cooked (⅔ cup) 21.0
Wheaties (1 cup) 23.0
Whole meal, cooked (1 cup) 40.0
Cervelat (4 ounces) 2.0
Champagne (see separate listing, page 103)
Chard, leaves (1 cup cooked) 1.6
Chard, leaves and stalks (1 cup cooked) 6.4
Cheese
American (1 ounce) 6
American, grated (1 tablespoon) 1
Bleu (1 ounce) 6
Bleu, domestic (1 ounce) 6
Brie (1 ounce) 5
Camembert (1 ounce) 5
Chateau (1 ounce) 1.1
Cheddar (1 ounce) 6
Cheddar, grated (1 tablespoon) 1
Cheddar, processed (1 slice) 6
Cheese food (1 ounce) 3
Cottage (1 cup) 4.5
Cottage (1 ounce) 6
Cottage, creamed (1 cup) 5.7
Cream (1 ounce) 6
Cream (1 tablespoon) 3

Edam (1 ounce) 1.1

Feta (1 ounce) 5

Gorgonzola (1 ounce) 5

Gruyere (1 ounce) 5

Liederkranz (1 ounce) 6

Limburger (1 ounce) 6

Mysost (1 ounce) 15.4

Neufchatel (1 ounce) 2.2

Pabst-ett (1 ounce) 2.2

Parmesan (1 ounce) 7

Parmesan, grated (1 tablespoon) 2

Pimiento (1 ounce) 1.9

Pot (3 ounces) 1.8

Provolone (1 ounce) 8

Roquefort (1 ounce) 5

Swiss, natural (1 ounce) 5

Swiss, processed (1 ounce) 5

Velveeta (1 ounce) 3.0

Cheese fondue (3½ ounces) 10.8

Cheese sauce (see Sauces)

Cheese soufflé (½ cup) 6.8

Cheese spread

Bacon (1 ounce) 1.9

Old English (1 ounce) 1.9

Olive pimiento (1 ounce) 1.9

Pimiento (1 ounce) 1.9

Pineapple (1 ounce) 2.9

Relish (1 ounce) 3.0
Roka bleu (1 ounce) 1.9
Cheese straws (3) 3.0
Cheesecake (see Cakes)
Cherries
    Fresh, sour or sweet (15 large or 25 small) 14.8
    Fresh, pitted (1 cup) 19.7
    Candied (1 large) 4.3
    Canned, Bing, low calorie (1 cup) 22.0
    Canned, Bing, in syrup (1 cup) 59.0
    Canned, red sour, water pack (1 cup) 23.8
    Canned, red sour, in syrup (1 cup) 56.6
    Canned, Royal Anne, in syrup (1 cup) 48.8
    Canned, Royal Anne, low calorie (1 cup) 21.0
    Maraschino (1) 5.2
Chestnuts (2 large) 7.2
Chewing gum (see Gum)
Chicken
    Boiled 0
    Broiler 0
    Canned, boned 0
    Creamed (½ cup) 5.7
    Fryer 0
    Fryer (½ bird, fried with flour) 6.2
    Fryer (small leg, fried with flour) 1.5
    Gizzard 0
    Heart (see Heart)

Liver (see Liver)

Potted 0

Roaster 0

Stewing 0

Chicken à la king (½ cup) 6.6

Chicken broth (see Soups)

Chicken croquettes (see Croquettes)

Chicken fat (see Fats)

Chicken paprikash (small serving) 5.7

Chicken pot pie, frozen (8 ounces) 50.4

Chicken salad (see Salads)

Chicken soup (see Soups)

Chicken TV dinner (1) 41.5

Chick-peas (½ cup, dry) 64.0

Chicory (10 small leaves) 1.0

Chili con carne (½ cup without beans) 6.6

Chili con carne (½ cup with beans) 14.0

Chili powder (1 tablespoon) 5

Chili sauce (see Sauces)

Chinese cabbage (see Cabbage)

Chipped beef (see Beef)

Chives (1 tablespoon chopped) ....trace

Chocolate beverage, with milk (1 cup) 17.1

Chocolate cake (see Cakes)

Chocolate candy (see Candies)

Chocolate ice cream (see Ice Cream)

Chocolate malted (see Milkshake)

Chocolate milk (see Milk)

Chocolate milkshake (see Milkshake)

Chocolate pudding (see Puddings)

Chocolate sauce (see Sauces)

Chocolate syrup (see Syrups)

Chop suey, with meat, canned (1 cup) 9.6

Chow-chow (see Pickles)

Chow mein, chicken, canned, without noodles (1 cup)16.1

Chutney, apple (5 tablespoons) 52.3

Chutney, tomato (5 tablespoons) 38.8

Cider, fermented (see separate listing, page 95)

Cider, sweet (1 cup) 25.8

Cinnamon bun (see Buns)

Clam chowder (see Soups)

Clam cocktail (4 clams, 1 tablespoon sauce) 4.5

Clam dip, sour cream (3 teaspoons) 5

Clams

    Raw, meat only (5-10) 3.4

    Cherry stone (6) 4.5

    Littleneck (6) 4.5

    Steamers (6) 4.4

    Canned (3 ounces, drained) 1.6

    Canned (3 ounces with liquid) 2.2

    Fried with batter (6) 9.5

    Steamed (6 with 1 tablespoon butter) 4.6

    Stuffed, baked (2) 9.5

Club sandwich, (see Sandwiches)

Coca Cola (see Soft drinks)

Cocoa, all milk (1 cup) 24.8

Cocoa, ½ milk, ½ water (¾ cup) 12.6

Cocoa, skim milk (¾ cup) 17.2

Cocoa powder (1 cup) 81.6

Cocoa powder (1 tablespoon) 5.0

Cocoamalt, all milk (1 cup) 33.5

Coconut, fresh (2-inch square) 6.3

Coconut, fresh, shredded (1 cup) 13.2

Coconut, dried, shredded, sweetened (1 cup) 33.0

Coconut custard pie (see Pies)

Coconut milk (see Milk)

Codfish 0

Codfish, creamed (½ cup) 8.1

Codfish balls or cakes (2) 9.6

Coffee, black (1 cup) 8

Coffee with 1 tablespoon light cream 1.3

Coffee with 1 tablespoon evaporated milk 2.3

Coffee with 1 tablespoon heavy cream 1.2

Coffee with 1 tablespoon condensed milk 11.1

Coffee with 1 tablespoon milk 1.5

Coffee with 1 tablespoon skim milk 1.6

Coffee with 1 teaspoon sugar 4.8

Coffee cake (see Cakes)

Collards (½ cup cooked) 6.9

Consommé (see Soups)

Cookies

Animal Crackers (1) 1.5

Arrowroot (1) 3.6

Brownies (1) 16.2

Butter (1) 6.9

Butterscotch (1) 14.6

Chocolate (1) 6.0

Chocolate chip (1) 7.8

Chocolate marshmallow (1) 8.6

Chocolate wafer (1) 6.0

Coconut bar (1) 9.4

Date (1) 25.8

Devils Food squares (1) 11.8

Iced (1) 10.1

Fig bar (1) 11.4

Gaiety Creme Sandwich (1) 14.0

Gaiety Creme Sandwich, chocolate (1) 15.6

Gingersnap (1) 3.2

Gingersnap (1 large) 10.0

Graham cracker (1) 5.3

Graham cracker, chocolate covered (1) 6.9

Hermit (1) 6.9

Lady finger (1) 6.2

Lorna Doone (1) 5.4

Macaroon (1) 14.3

Molasses (1) 5.0

Nabisco Devil (1) 11.8

Oatmeal (1 large) 17.0

Oreo Creme Sandwich (1) 8.7
Peanut (1) 7.3
Plain (1 large) 6.9
Raisin (1) 12.9
Scotch shortbread (1) 5.4
Social Tea (1) 3.8
Sugar (1) 6.9
Sugar wafer (1) 1.5
Toll House (1) 7.2
Vanilla wafer (1) 3.6
Waffle creams (1) 7.2
Cooking fat (see Fats)
Corn (1 ear) 21.0
Corn (1 cup kernels) 37.6
Corn, canned (1 cup kernels with liquid) 51.2
Corn, frozen (½ cup kernels) 17.6
Corn bread (see Breads)
Corn flakes (see Cereals)
Corn fritter (1) 10.2
Corn grits (¼ cup dry) 28.4
Corn grits (1 cup cooked) 26.6
Corn muffins (see Muffins)
Corn oil (see Oils)
Corn pudding, Southern (½ cup) 13.4
Corn syrup (see Syrups)
Corned beef (see Beef)
Cornmeal (¼ cup dry) 28.9

Cornmeal (1 cup cooked) 25.5
Cornstarch (1 tablespoon) 7.0
Cornstarch pudding (see Puddings)
Cottage cheese (see Cheese)
Cowpeas (1 cup cooked) 25.4
Crab (1 pound meat) 2.3
Crab, canned (8 ounces) 2.5
Crab, deviled (1 medium) 9.7
Crab, soft-shell, fried, with batter (1 small) 8.6
Crab apple (1) 3.5
Crab Jambalaya (1 serving) 15.8
Crab paste (1 teaspoon) 1
Crab salad (see Salads)
Cracker meal (1 tablespoon) 7.3
Crackers
    Animal (see Cookies)
    Blue cheese (1) 1.4
    Butter thins (1) 2.8
    Cheese tidbits (15 tiny) 3.0
    Graham (see Cookies)
    Holland rusk (see Toast)
    Matzoth (1 6-inch piece) 17.5
    Melba toast (see Toast)
    Oyster (10) 7.1
    Peanut butter-cheese sandwich (1) 4.5
    Pretzels (see Pretzels)
    Ritz (1) 2.1

Rye thins (1) 1.9

Ry-Krisp (1 double square) 9.6

Saltine (1) 2.9

Soda (1) 4.4

Triscuit (1) 2.9

Uneeda (1) 3.9

Water (1) 6.9

Wheat (1) 4.4

Wheat thins (1) 1.3

Zwieback (see Toast)

Cranberries, fresh (1 cup) 10.8

Cranberry juice (see Juices)

Cranberry relish, with orange (¼ cup) 25.0

Cranberry sauce (see Sauces)

Cream

Light (½ pint) 8.2

Light (1 tablespoon) 5

Half and half (see Milk)

Heavy (½ pint) 7.2

Heavy (1 tablespoon) 4

Sour (1 cup) ....,...7.7

Whipped (½ pint) 3.6

Whipped (1 tablespoon) 2

Cream cheese (see Cheese)

Cream soup (see Soups)

Crème de menthe (see separate listing, page 103)

Creole sauce (see Sauces)

Cress, garden (1 pound) 15.0

Cress, garden (1 cup cooked) 9.6

Cress, water (1 pound) 15.2

Cress, water (1 bunch) 3.3

Cress, water (10 sprigs) 5

Crisco 0

Croquettes, beef (1 medium) 8.8

Croquettes, chicken (1 medium) 8.8

Croquettes, fish (1 medium) 8.8

Croquettes, potato (1 medium) 16.7

Croutons (½-inch cube) 6

Cucumber pickles (see Pickles)

Cucumbers (1 medium) 2.8

Cucumbers (6 slices) 1.4

Cupcake (see Cakes)

Curaçao (see separate listing, page 103)

Currant jelly (see Jams, jellies)

Currants (1 cup) 17.0

Currants, dried, sweetened (1 cup) 142.4

Curry powder (1 teaspoon) 5

Custard (see Puddings)

Custard pie (see Pies)

grams

Daiquiri (see separate listing, page 101)

Dandelion greens (1 pound) 40.0

Dandelion greens (½ cup cooked) 8.0

Danish pastry (see Pastries)

Date torte (see Cakes)

Dates (1 cup pitted) 134.0

Dates (3 or 4) 22.6

Deviled meat (1 tablespoon) .... trace

Dextromaltose (1 tablespoon) 6.8

Dill pickles (see Pickles)

Divinity (see Candies)

Doughnuts

    Cake, plain (1) 17.5

    Cruller, sugared (1) 20.0

    Jelly (1) 30.0

    Raised or yeast (1) 13.7

    Sugared or iced (1) 21.7

Dry milk (see Milk)

Duck 0

Duck eggs (see Eggs)

E

Eclair (see Pastries)

Eels 0

Eels, smoked 0

Egg foo yung (1 serving) 6.5

Egg roll (1) 3.5

Eggnog, alcoholic (see separate listing, page 101)

Eggnog, all milk (1 cup) 24.7

Eggplant (½ cup) 5.5

Eggplant, fried with batter (1 slice) 11.5

Eggs

    Raw (1 medium) 3

    Raw, whites (1) 2

    Raw, yolks (1) 1

    Boiled or poached (1 medium) 3

    Creamed (2 eggs, 3 tablespoons sauce) 5.1

    Deviled (1) 5

    Dried (1 tablespoon) 2

    Dried (1 cup) 2.7

    Duck (1 large) 2.4

    Fried, in butter (1 medium) 4

Omelet, plain in butter (1 egg) 4
Omelet, cheese (2 eggs) 9
Omelet, Spanish (2 eggs) 7.6
Scrambled, with milk (1) 1.0
Endive (2 stalks) 4.0
Endive (10 inner leaves) 1.0
Escarole (2 large leaves) 2.0
Escarole (7 small leaves) 8

grams

Fats

Bacon (1 tablespoon) 0
Chicken 0
Cooking 0
Ghee (3½ ounces) 0
Vegetable 0
Fennel leaves (2 pieces) 2.0
Fig bars (see Cookies)
Figs

Fresh (2 small) 19.6
Canned (1 cup with syrup) 79.6

Canned (3 with 2 tablespoons syrup) 36.0

Canned, low calorie (½ cup) 10.0

Dried (1 large) 13.6

Dried (1 cup cut) 64.4

Kadota (3, 1 tablespoon juice) 10.0

Filberts (10 to 12) 2.6

Finnan haddie 0

Finnan haddie, creamed (4 ounces) 6.1

Fish (see individual listings)

Fish, creamed (½ cup) 6.1

Fish cakes (1) 9.4

Fish croquettes (see Croquettes)

Fish chowder (see Soups)

Fish sticks, breaded, frozen (4 ounces) 7.5

Flounder 0

Flour

Buckwheat (1 cup) 70.6

Cake (1 cup) 72.2

Corn (1 cup) 84.6

Rye (1 cup) 62.3

Soybean (1 cup) 38.1

Wheat (1 cup) 83.7

White (1 cup) 83.7

White (1 tablespoon) 5.4

Fondant (see Candies)

Frankfurters (1 cooked, about 1.8 ounces) 1.0

French bread (see Breads)

French dressing (see Salad dressings)

French pastry (see Pastries)

French toast, without syrup (1 piece) 12.2

French toast, 1 tablespoon corn syrup (1 piece) 27.2

French toast, 1 tablespoon maple syrup (1 piece) ..25.0

Frog legs 0

Frog legs, fried with batter (2) 4.0

Fruit (see individual listings)

Fruit cake (see Cakes)

Fruit cocktail, fresh (1 cup) 34.2

Fruit cocktail, canned (1 cup with syrup) 47.6

Fruit cocktail, canned, low calorie (1 cup) 9.3

Fruit salad (see Salads)

Fruits for salad, canned (3 tablespoons) 29.0

Fruits for salad, canned, low calorie (⅔ cup) 7.0

Fruits, glazed (see Candies)

Fudge (see Candies)

Fudge sundae (see ice cream sundaes)

grams

Garbanzos (see Chick-peas)

Garden cress (see Cress)

Garlic (1 clove) 4

Gefilte fish (4 ounces) 9.6

Gelatin, dry, plain 0

Gelatin, fruit flavors, prepared (½ cup) 18.0

Gelatin, fruit flavors, fruit added (½ cup) 26.8

Gelatin salad (see Salads)

Gin (see separate listing, page 102)

Ginger ale (see Soft drinks)

Ginger root (3½ ounces) 6.9

Ginger root, candied (1 ounce) 24.7

Gingerbread (see Cakes)

Gingersnaps (see Cookies)

Glazed fruit (see Candies)

Goat's milk (see Milk)

Goose 0

Gooseberries (1 cup) 12.9

Goulash, Hungarian (½ cup) 9.5

Graham crackers (see Cookies)

Grape juice (see Juices)
Grape Nuts (see Cereals)
Grape soda (see Soft drinks)
Grapefruit
    Fresh (½ large) 22.2
    Fresh (½ medium) 18.2
    Fresh (½ small) 14.0
    Fresh (1 cup sections) 19.6
    Fresh, pink (½ medium) 18.2
    Canned (1 cup with syrup) 42.6
    Canned, water pack (1 cup with liquid) 19.2
Grapefruit juice (see Juices)
Grapes
    Fresh, American type (1 cup) 18.5
    (Concord, Delaware, Niagara)
    Fresh, European type (1 cup) 25.9
    (Malaga, Muscat, Tokay)
    Thompson seedless (½ cup) 16.7
    Canned (1 cup with syrup) 45.4
    Canned, water pack (1 cup) 22.0
Gravy (¼ cup) 4.2
Green beans (see Beans, green)
Green onions (see Onions, green)
Green pea soup (see Soups)
Griddle cakes (see Pancakes)
Grits, hominy (½ cup cooked) 13.3
Guava (1) 17.1

Guava butter (see Jams, jellies)
Guava jelly (see Jams, jellies)
Guinea hen 0
Gum, chewing (1 stick) 1.7
Gum, chewing, candy coated (2 pieces) 2.5
Gumbo soup (see Soups)

grams

Haddock 0
Haddock, creamed (4 ounces) 6.1
Haddock, fried with flour (1 fillet, about 3 oz.) 8.1
Halibut, broiled 0
Halibut, creamed (4 ounces) 6.1
Ham
    Fresh 0
    Baked, cured (3 ounces, no bone) 3
    Boiled 0
    Canned, boneless (3 ounces) 4
    Canned, deviled (1 tablespoon) 2
    Canned, spiced (2 ounces) 2
    Hock (3 ounces) 0

Prosciutto (1½ ounces) 0

Smoked, cooked 0

Ham sandwich (see Sandwiches)

Hamburger (see Beef)

Hamburger sandwich (see Sandwiches)

Hard candy (see Candies)

Hard sauce (see Sauces)

Hash, beef (1 cup) 19.0

Hash, canned corned beef, with potatoes (1 cup) ...24.3

Hash, turkey (1 cup) 19.0

Hazelnuts (10-12) 3.0

Head cheese (3 ounces) 0

Heart, beef, lean (3 ounces) 7

Heart, beef, braised (3 ounces) 8

Heart, chicken (3 ounces) 1.3

Heart, chicken (9 or 10) 1.6

Heart, pork (3 ounces) 4

Herbs (1 teaspoon) 0

Hermits (see Cookies)

Herring

    Atlantic 0

    Canned, in tomato sauce (8 oz.) 8.4

    Lake 0

    Pacific 0

    Kippered 0

    Marinated with cream (small piece) 8

    Pickled 0

Smoked 0
Hershey bar (see Candies)
Hickory nuts (15 small) 2.0
Highball (see separate listing, page 102)
Holland rusk (see Toast)
Hollandaise (see Sauces)
Hominy grits (see Grits)
Honey (see Syrups)
Honeydew melon (1 wedge) 12.8
Horsemeat 0
Horseradish (1 tablespoon) 4
Hot dog (see Sandwiches, Frankfurter)
Hubbard squash (see Squash)
Huckleberries (1 cup) 21.1

I

grams

Ice cream
    Plain, vanilla (¼ pint) 15.1
    Chocolate (¼ pint) 16.6
    Coffee (¼ pint) 15.6
    Frozen custard (¼ pint) 16.3

Peach (¼ pint) 15.9
Sherbet, with milk (¼ pint) 44.0
Sherbet, with water (see Ice Cream, ices)
Strawberry (¼ pint) 15.9
Ice cream, ices (¼ pint) 35.2
Ice cream, milk (¼ pint) 21.2
Ice cream cone (cone alone) 3.5
Ice cream parfait, coffee (1) 14.4
Ice cream parfait, maple (1) 19.9
Ice cream pop, chocolate covered 14.5
Ice pop (twin) 23.7
Ice cream soda
Chocolate, vanilla ice cream (10-oz.) 47.9
Chocolate, chocolate ice cream (10-oz.) 48.7
Strawberry, strawberry ice cream (10-oz.) 48.2
Vanilla, vanilla ice cream (10-oz.) 47.1
Ice cream sundae
Banana split 92.5
Butterscotch 55.6
Chocolate (vanilla ice cream) 52.8
Chocolate (chocolate ice cream) 54.3
Hot fudge 52.8
Ice milk (see Ice cream, milk)
Ice water (see Ice cream, ices)
Indian pudding (see Puddings)
Irish whiskey (see separate listing, page 102)
Italian bread (see Breads)

J

grams

Jams, jellies

    Blackberry jam (1 tablespoon) 14.2

    Blackberry jelly (1 tablespoon) 13.0

    Cranberry jelly (1 tablespoon) 8.6

    Currant jelly (1 tablespoon) 13.0

    Guava butter (1 tablespoon) 10.0

    Guava jelly (1 tablespoon) 13.0

    Grape jelly (1 tablespoon) 13.0

    Lemon jelly (1 tablespoon) 13.0

    Orange marmalade (1 tablespoon) 14.0

    Papaya marmalade (1 tablespoon) 14.6

    Plum jam (1 tablespoon) 14.2

    Preserves (1 tablespoon) 14.2

    Strawberry jam (1 tablespoon) 14.2

Jell-O (see Gelatin)

Juices

    Apple, fresh or canned (1 cup) 34.2

    Apricot juice, unsweetened (1 cup) 29.2

    Apricot nectar (1 cup) 36.2

    Blackberry (1 cup) 18.0

Blueberry (1 cup) 32.4
Carrot (1 cup) 12.8
Cider (see Cider)
Cranberry (1 cup) 36.0
Currant, black (1 cup) 34.4
Currant, red (1 cup) 25.2
Grape (1 cup) 42.0
Grape, frozen, sweetened (1 cup) 31.0
Grapefruit (1 cup) 23.0
Grapefruit, canned, unsweetened (1 cup) 24.0
Grapefruit, canned, sweetened (1 cup) 30.4
Grapefruit, frozen, unswtd. (6-oz. can) 72.0
Grapefruit, frozen, unswtd. diluted (1 cup) 24.1
Grapefruit, frozen, sweetened (6-oz. can) 85.0
Grapefruit, frozen, swtd., diluted (1 cup) 28.0
Lemon (1 cup) 18.9
Lemon (1 tablespoon) 1.2
Lime (1 cup) 20.4
Lime (1 tablespoon) 1.2
Loganberry (1 cup) 24.8
Nectarine (1 cup) 34.9
Orange, California Valencia (1 cup) 27.0
Orange, Florida early season (1 cup) 23.0
Orange, Florida late season (1 cup) 27.0
Orange, canned, unsweetened (1 cup) 27.0
Orange, canned, sweetened (1 cup) 32.0
Orange, frozen, unsweetened (6-ounce can) ...80.0

Orange, frozen, unsweetened, diluted (1 cup) . . 24.4

Orange, dehydrated (4 ounces crystals) 100.0

Orange, dehydrated, water added (1 cup) 24.7

Orange-grapefruit, canned, unswtd. (1 cup) 23.6

Orange-grapefruit, canned, swtd. (1 cup) 28.0

Orange-grapefruit, frozen (6-ounce can) 77.7

Orange-grapefruit, frozen, diluted (1 cup) 24.0

Papaya (1 cup) 30.2

Peach nectar, canned (1 cup) 31.0

Pear nectar, canned (1 cup) 32.0

Pineapple, frozen, unsweetened (1 cup) 31.2

Pineapple, canned (1 cup) 32.4

Pomegranate (1 cup) 18.2

Prune, canned (1 cup) 45.6

Raspberry (1 cup) 25.6

Sauerkraut (1 cup) 6.0

Tangerine, canned, sweetened (1 cup) 27.0

Tangerine, canned, unsweetened (1 cup) 25.0

Tangerine, frozen (6-ounce can) 80.0

Tangerine, frozen, diluted (1 cup) 25.0

Tomato, canned (1 cup) 10.4

Vegetable, canned (1 cup) 8.6

V-8 (1 cup) 8.6

Junket (see Puddings)

K

	grams
Kale (1 cup cooked) 7.2
Kale, frozen (3½ ounces) 5.4

Kellogg's cereal (see Cereals)

Kidney beans (see Beans)

Kidneys

    Beef (½ cup) 9

    Lamb (½ cup) 1.0

    Pork (½ cup) 8

    Veal (½ cup) 9

Kippered herring (see Herring)

Kix (see Cereals)

Kohlrabi (⅔ cup diced) 6.7

Kohlrabi (1 cup cooked) 10.0

Kohlrabi, frozen (1 cup) 10.4

Krispies (see Cereals)

Kumquats (5 or 6) 9.7

L

	grams
Lady fingers (see Cookies)	
Lamb	
Breast	.0
Chops	.0
Ground	.0
Kidney (see Kidneys)	
Liver (see Liver)	
Roast, leg	.0
Roast, shoulder	.0
Lamb curry, with rice (½ cup)	22.9
Lamb shish kebab	.0
Lamb stew (see Stew)	
Lambsquarter or pigweed (½ cup)	8.3
Lard	.0
Layer cake (see Cakes)	
Leeks (3 medium)	7.9
Lemon (1 medium)	8.4
Lemon drops (see Candies)	
Lemon ice (see Ice cream, ices)	
Lemon jelly (see Jams, jellies)	

Lemon juice (see Juices)

Lemon peel, candied (see Candied peel)

Lemon pie (see Pies)

Lemon pudding (see Puddings)

Lemon sauce (see Sauces)

Lemon soda (see Soft drinks)

Lemonade, frozen concentrate (6-ounce can) 112.0

Lemonade, frozen, diluted (1 cup) 28.0

Lentil soup (see Soups)

Lentils (½ cup) 18.1

Lettuce (1 compact head) 13.0

Lettuce (1 cup) 2.9

Lettuce (4 small leaves) 1.0

Lettuce and tomato salad (see Salads)

Lichee nuts (6) 10.5

Lichee nuts, dried (3½ ounces) 52.5

Liederkranz cheese (see Cheese)

Lifesavers (see Candies)

Limburger cheese (see Cheese)

Lime (1 large) 9.0

Lime juice (see Juices)

Limeade, frozen concentrate (6-oz. can) 108.0

Limeade, frozen, diluted (1 cup) 27.0

Liquid diets (1 day) 110.0

Liver

    Beef (3½ ounces) 6.0

    Calves' (3½ ounces) 4.0

Canned, strained (1 jar, 3½ ounces) 1.8

Chicken (3 ounces) 3.0

Chicken (1 medium) 1.0

Chopped (3 ounces) 3.0

Goose (2 medium) 4.0

Goose liver paste (see Pâté de foie gras)

Lamb (1 slice) 4.3

Pork (1 slice) 3.8

Liver loaf (1 slice) 9.4

Liver spread (2 tablespoons) 2

Liverwurst (1 slice) 5

Liverwurst sandwich (see Sandwiches)

Lobster

Fresh, (1 pound in shell) 6

Baked or broiled 6

Broiled (1 African tail, about ½ lb.) 3

Canned or cooked (½ cup meat) 7

Creamed (½ cup) 6.4

Lobster Cantonese (1 serving) 7.5

Lobster cocktail (½ cup meat, 2 tbs. sauce) 3.0

Lobster cocktail (½ cup meat, wedge lemon) 8

Lobster cocktail (½ cup meat, mayonnaise) 9

Lobster Newburgh (½ cup) 7.7

Lobster paste (1 teaspoon) 1

Lobster salad (see Salads)

Lobster Thermidor (1 lobster) 14.8

Loganberries (⅔ cup) 15.0

Loganberries, canned (1 cup) 25.0

Loganberry juice (see Juices)

Lollipops (see Candies)

Lotus root (⅔ average segment) 15.7

Lox 0

Luncheon meat (1 ounce) 5

Luncheon meat sandwich (see Sandwiches)

M

	grams

Macadamia nuts (10 to 12) 1.5

Macaroni, cooked 8-10 minutes (1 cup) 39.0

Macaroni, cooked till tender (1 cup) 32.0

Macaroni and cheese (1 cup) 44.0

Macaroni salad (see Salads)

Macaroons (see Cookies)

Mackerel 0

Madeira wine (see separate listing, page 103)

Malted milk (see Milkshake)

Malted milk powder (1 tablespoon) 6.8

Maltex cereal (see Cereals)

Mandarin orange (see Tangerines)

Mango (1 medium) 34.5

Manhattan cocktail (see separate listing, page 101)

Maple syrup (see Syrups)

Margarine (1 cup) 1.8

Margarine (1 tablespoon) 1

Margarine (1 pat) ....trace

Marmalade (see Jams, jellies)

Mars candy (see Candies)

Marshmallow (see Candies)

Marshmallow sauce (see Sauces)

Martini cocktail (see separate listing, page 101)

Mashed potatoes (see Potatoes)

Matzoth (see Crackers)

Mayonnaise (see Salad dressings)

Maypo oat cereal (see Cereals)

Meal, cracker (see Cracker meal)

Meat (see individual listings)

Meat croquette (see Croquettes, beef)

Meat gravy (see Gravy)

Meat loaf, beef-pork (1 slice) 11.5

Meat stew (see Stew)

Melba toast (see Toast)

Melon balls, frozen (1 cup) 12.5

Melons (see individual listings)

Meringue (¼ cup) 8.3

Milk

     Whole (1 cup) 11.8

Whole (1 tablespoon) 7
Skim, nonfat (1 cup) 13.0
Buttermilk (1 cup) 12.4
Canned, evaporated (1 cup) 24.0
Canned, evaporated (1 tablespoon) 1.5
Canned, sweetened condensed (1 cup) 170.0
Canned, sweetened condensed (1 tablespoon) ..10.3
Chocolate flavored (1 cup) 27.9
Chocolate flavored, skim (1 cup) 28.1
Cocoa (see Cocoa)
Coconut (1 cup) 12.0
Dry, whole (1 cup) 39.0
Dry, whole (1 tablespoon) 2.4
Dry, nonfat (1 cup) 42.0
Dry, nonfat (1 tablespoon) 2.7
Goat's (1 cup) 11.2
Half and half (1 cup) 11.0
Malted (see Milkshake)
Milkshake, chocolate (10 ounces) 57.0
Milkshake, chocolate malted (10 ounces) 70.0
Mincemeat pie (see Pies)
Mineral oil (see Oils)
Mint (1 teaspoon chopped) 0
Mint julep (see separate listing, page 58)
Mints (see Candies)
Mixed vegetables (see Vegetables, mixed)
Molasses (see Syrups)

Muffins

Blueberry (1 small) 23.2

Bran (1 medium) 20.5

Corn (1 medium) 18.0

Date (1 medium) 40.8

Egg (1 medium) 20.2

English (1 medium) 17.5

Raisin (1 medium) 27.2

Soy (1 medium) 16.7

White (1 medium) 17.1

Whole wheat (1 medium) 17.1

Muscatel wine (see separate listing, page 103)

Mushroom soup (see Soups)

Mushrooms, raw (½ pound) 9.7

Mushrooms, raw (4 large or 10 medium) 4.0

Mushrooms, canned (1 cup with liquid) 9.0

Mushrooms, sautéed (7 small) 2.8

Muskmelon (½ medium) 8.3

Mussels (1 pound) 7.2

Mussels, smoked (1) ....trace

Mustard, dry 0

Mustard, prepared (1 tablespoon) 8

Mustard greens (1 pound) 13.2

Mustard greens (1 cup cooked) 5.8

Mutton 0

grams

Nabisco wafers (see Cookies)
Navy beans (see Beans, navy)
Nectar (see Juices)
Nectarines (2 medium) 16.0
Noodle soup (see Soups)
Noodles, egg (1 cup cooked) 37.0
Noodles, fried, canned (1 ounce) 16.7
Nuts (see individual listings)
Nuts, mixed (8 to 12) 2.7

grams

Oatmeal (see Cereals)
Oatmeal cookies (see Cookies)
Ocean perch (see Perch)

Oils

    Corn 0

    Cottonseed 0

    Mineral 0

    Olive 0

    Palm, red unrefined 0

    Peanut 0

    Salad 0

Okra (8 pods cooked) 6.3

Old Fashioned (see separate listing, page 101)

Oleomargarine (see Margarine)

Olive cheese spread (see Cheese spreads)

Olive oil (see Oils)

Olives, green (10 large) 1.0

Olives, ripe or black (10 large) 2.0

Omelet (see Eggs)

Onion soup (see Soups)

Onions

    Raw (1 medium) 10.5

    Raw (1 tablespoon chopped) 1.0

    Cooked (1 cup) 18.0

    Dehydrated (2 tablespoons) 8.0

    Green (6 small) 5.3

    Scalloped (½ cup) 15.2

Orange ice (see Ice cream, ices)

Orange juice (see Juices)

Orange soda (see Soft drinks)

Oranges

    Fresh (1 large) 26.0

    Fresh (1 medium) 17.0

    Fresh (1 small) 11.5

    Fresh (1 cup sections) 22.0

Ovaltine (1 cup) 21.7

Oyster stew (1 cup, 6-8 oysters) 11.0

Oyster stew, frozen (1 can) 19.6

Oysters

    Raw, meat only (5 to 8 medium) 5.6

    Fried with batter (6) 18.2

    Scalloped (6) 31.6

grams

Pablum (see Cereals)

Pancakes, buckwheat (1 4-inch cake) 10.7

Pancakes, white flour (1 4-inch cake) 12.9

Papaya (1 cup cubes) 18.0

Papaya juice (see Juices)

Parfait (see Ice cream parfait)

Parmesan cheese (see Cheeses)

Parsley (1 tablespoon chopped) 2

Parsnips (½ cup cooked) 10.8

Passion fruit (½ cup) 14.0

Pasta (see individual listings)

Pastrami 0

Pastries

    Cream puff (1) 15.7

    Danish (1 medium) 22.8

    Doughnuts (see Doughnuts)

    Eclair, chocolate, custard (1) 20.3

    Eclair, chocolate, cream (1) 15.7

    French pastry (medium) 15.0-40.0

    Petit fours (1) 25.0

Pâté de foie gras (1 tablespoon) 7

Pea soup (see Soups)

Peaches

    Fresh (1 medium) 9.7

    Fresh (1 cup slices) 16.0

    Canned (1 cup with syrup) 49.0

    Canned, water pack (1 cup with liquid) 17.0

    Canned, strained (1 ounce) 5.0

    Dried (1 cup) 109.0

    Dried, cooked, unswtd. (1 cup with liquid) 58.0

    Dried, cooked, sweetened (1 cup with liquid) ...94.0

    Frozen, sliced, sweetened (1 cup) 56.0

Peanut brittle (see Candies)

Peanut butter (1 tablespoon) 3.4

Peanut butter sandwich (see Sandwiches)

Peanuts (1 cup halves) 34.0

Peanuts (18 to 20) 4.2

Peanuts (1 tablespoon chopped) 2.1

Pears

    Fresh (1) 23.9

    Fresh (1 cup quarters) 31.8

    Canned (1 cup with syrup) 49.2

    Canned (2 halves with 2 tablespoons syrup) 23.0

    Canned, water pack (1 cup with liquid) 19.8

    Canned, low calorie (1 cup) 14.4

    Canned, strained (1 ounce) 4.5

Peas

    Fresh (1 cup cooked) 19.0

    Fresh (1 pound, in pod) 36.1

    Canned (1 cup with liquid) 32.2

    Canned (1 cup, drained) 27.6

    Canned, strained (1 ounce) 2.0

    Dried (½ cup cooked) 18.1

    Frozen (½ cup) 11.3

    Split (1 cup cooked) 45.0

Peas, edible pods (see Snow peas)

Pecans (12 nutmeats) 1.8

Pecans, chopped (1 tablespoon) 9

Pecans (1 cup halves) 14.6

Pepperpot soup (see Soups)

Peppers, green (1 medium) 3.0

Peppers, green, chopped (1 tablespoon) 5
Peppers, green, stuffed (1 medium) 12.2
Peppers, red, hot dried (1 tablespoon) 9.0
Peppers, red (1 medium) 4.0
Pepsi Cola (see Soft drinks)
Perch, fresh 0
Perch, fried with batter (3 ounces) 6.0
Persian melon (1 wedge) 12.8
Persimmons (1 medium) 20.0
Pheasant 0
Pickle relish (1 tablespoon) 3.4
Pickle relish, mustard (1 tablespoon) 3.6
Pickles, chow-chow (4 pieces) 1.1
Pickles, cucumber, bread and butter (4 slices) 5.1
Pickles, cucumber (6 slices) 7
Pickles, dill (1 large) 3.0
Pickles, sour (1 large) 3.0
Pickles, sweet (1 medium) 2.6
Pie crust (double crust) 143.0
Pie crust (bottom crust) 72.0
Pie crust, graham cracker (bottom crust) 64.4
Pies (all pieces ⅛ of 9-inch pie)
    Apple (1 piece) 46.7
    Apricot (1 piece) 57.7
    Banana cream (1 piece) 35.9
    Berry (1 piece) 43.0
    Blackberry (1 piece) 43.0

Blueberry (1 piece) 44.0

Butterscotch, whipped cream (1 piece) 42.1

Cherry (1 piece) 47.7

Chocolate chiffon, whipped cream (1 piece) 33.2

Chocolate meringue (1 piece) 32.3

Coconut custard (1 piece) 30.0

Cream (1 piece) 41.7

Custard (1 piece) 29.9

Lemon chiffon (1 piece) 35.2

Lemon meringue (1 piece) 39.3

Mincemeat (1 piece) 53.9

Peach (1 piece) 58.0

Peach, whipped cream (1 piece) 59.0

Pecan (1 piece) 57.6

Pineapple (1 piece) 36.0

Pineapple-cheese (1 piece) 38.2

Pineapple cream (1 piece) 47.5

Pizza (see Pizza pie)

Prune, whipped cream (1 piece) 53.7

Pumpkin (1 piece) 29.4

Raisin (1 piece) 59.1

Rhubarb (1 piece) 49.7

Shoofly (1 piece) 48.3

Strawberry (1 piece) 51.4

Strawberry cream (1 piece) 53.9

Pignolias (see Pine nuts)

Pig's feet 0

Pike 0

Pimiento, canned (1 medium) 2.2

Pimiento cheese (see Cheese)

Pine nuts, salted (½ cup) 5.6

Pine nuts, chopped (1 tablespoon) 7

Pineapple

    Fresh (1 cup diced) 19.0

    Fresh (1 slice) 11.5

    Canned (1 large slice with syrup) 26.0

    Canned (½ cup crushed) 27.5

    Canned, low calorie (½ cup) 11.0

    Candied (1 slice) 30.4

    Frozen (½ cup) 26.2

Pineapple cheese spread (see Cheese spreads)

Pineapple juice (see Juices)

Pistachio nuts (20) 1.6

Pistachio nuts, chopped (1 tablespoon) 1.5

Pistachio nuts, shelled (1 cup) 24.5

Pizza pie, with cheese (average piece) 25.2

Plantain (1) 44.3

Plums

    Fresh (1 medium) 7.0

    Canned (1 cup with syrup) 50.0

    Canned (6 halves with 2 tablespoons syrup) ...25.0

    Canned, low calorie (½ cup) 10.0

Poha, Hawaiian (1 cup) 11.3

Polish sausage (see Sausage)

Pomegranate (1 medium) 21.9

Pompano 0

Popcorn, no butter (1 cup popped) 11.0

Popcorn, sugar-coated (1 ounce) 24.1

Popover (1) 12.9

Porgy 0

Pork

    Chops 0

    Heart (see Heart)

    Kidney (see Kidneys)

    Liver (see Liver)

    Pig's feet (see Pig's feet)

    Roast 0

    Salt 0

    Sausage (see Sausage)

    Shoulder 0

    Sirloin 0

    Spareribs 0

    Tenderloin 0

Post Toasties (see Cereals)

Postum (1 teaspoon, dry) 8

Pot cheese (see Cheeses)

Pot roast (see Beef)

Potato chips (8 to 10) 10.0

Potato salad (see Salads)

Potato soup (see Soups)

Potatoes

Baked or boiled (1 medium) 21.0
Canned (3-4 small) 19.1
Creamed (½ cup) 14.1
French fried (10 pieces) 20.0
French fried, frozen (10 pieces) 15.0
Fried (½ cup) 30.9
Hash browned (1 cup) 62.2
Mashed, with milk (½ cup) 15.0
Mashed, with milk, butter (½ cup) 14.0
Scalloped (½ cup) 14.2
Potatoes, sweet
Raw (3½ ounces) 27.9
Baked (1) 36.0
Boiled (1) 39.0
Candied (1 small) 60.0
Canned (1 cup) 54.0
Dehydrated (3½ ounces) 84.5
Yam (1 cup cooked) 48.2
Yam, marshmallow topping (1 cup) 60.6
Poultry (see individual listings)
Poultry stuffing (see Stuffing)
Pound cake (see Cakes)
Preserves (see Jams, jellies)
Pretzels (1 very large) 12.7
Pretzels, 3-ring (1) 2.4
Pretzels (5 sticks or 1 small) 1.4
Prickly pear (1 medium) 4.6

Prosciutto (see Ham)
Prune juice (see Juices)
Prunes (4 medium) 19.0
Prunes, canned, strained (1 ounce) 7.0
Prunes, cooked, unsweetened (1 cup with liquid) 81.0
Prunes, cooked, sweetened (4-5) 31.2
Puddings
    Apple brown betty (½ cup) 35.2
    Apple dumpling (1) 54.0
    Apple snow (½ cup) 25.5
    Banana custard, with meringue (½ cup) 19.2
    Banana whip (½ cup) 15.5
    Bavarian, orange (1 serving) 39.8
    Blancmange (½ cup) 20.0
    Bread and butter (1 piece) 28.4
    Bread, with raisins (¾ cup) 47.8
    Butterscotch (½ cup) 28.9
    Butterscotch, sugar-free (½ cup) 8.9
    Caramel (½ cup) 28.9
    Chocolate (½ cup) 30.6
    Chocolate, skim milk (½ cup) 30.1
    Cornstarch, butterscotch (½ cup) 37.4
    Cornstarch, chocolate (½ cup) 37.1
    Cornstarch, vanilla (½ cup) 20.0
    Cottage pudding (1 piece) 43.8
    Cottage pudding, 2 tbs. lemon sauce (1 piece) .61.1
    Custard (½ cup) 14.0

Indian (⅔ cup) 22.6

Jell-O (see Gelatine)

Junket (½ cup) 12.2

Lemon sponge (1 serving) 26.5

Lemon sponge with custard sauce (1 serving) ..41.3

Prune whip (½ cup) 25.1

Rice, with eggs (½ cup) 16.8

Rice, with raisins (½ cup) 32.2

Tapioca (½ cup) 11.6

Tapioca, apricot (½ cup) 40.8

Tapioca, chocolate (½ cup) 32.5

Vanilla (½ cup) 23.8

Pumpkin (3½ ounces) 7.6

Pumpkin, canned (1 cup) 18.0

Pumpkin pie (see Pies)

Q

grams

Quail, broiled 0

Quince (1 medium) 10.2

Quinine water (see Soft drinks)

R

	grams
Rabbit	.0
Rabbit stew (see Stew)	
Radishes (4 small)	2.0
Radishes, Chinese (3½ ounces)	4.5
Raisin bread (see Breads)	
Raisin sauce (see Sauces)	
Raisins (1 cup)	124.0
Raisins (1 tablespoon)	4.5
Raisins (4)	3.2
Raisins, cooked, sweetened (½ cup)	35.9
Ralston (see Cereals)	
Raspberries, black (1 cup)	21.0
Raspberries, red (1 cup)	17.0
Raspberries, canned (1 cup with syrup)	53.6
Raspberries, canned, water pack (1 cup, liquid)	6.2
Raspberries, frozen (10-ounce carton)	70.0
Raspberries, frozen (3 ounces)	23.7
Raspberry juice (see Juices)	
Ravioli, cheese filling (4 squares, sauce)	24.4
Red snapper	.0

Relish (see Pickle relish)

Relish cheese spread (see Cheese spreads)

Rhubarb

    Raw (1 cup diced) 4.6

    Cooked, sweetened (1 cup) 98.0

    Canned, low calorie (1 cup) 4.6

    Frozen (½ cup) 22.9

Rhubarb pie (see Pies)

Rice, brown (1 cup cooked) 43.0

Rice, fried (1 cup) 44.0

Rice, white (1 cup cooked) 44.0

Rice, white, converted (1 cup cooked) 44.2

Rice, wild (1 cup cooked) 30.2

Rice, Spanish (¾ cup) 26.2

Rice Krispies (see Cereals)

Rice pudding (see Puddings)

Rice puffs (see Cereals)

Roka bleu cheese spread (see Cheese spreads)

Rolls

    Cloverleaf (1) 20.5

    Hamburger (1) 20.9

    Hard (1 large) 31.0

    Frankfurter (1) 20.5

    French (1) 20.9

    Onion (1 large) 31.0

    Parker House (1) 13.5

    Plain (1) 20.0

Sweet (1) 27.0
Whole wheat (1) 18.3
Romaine (1 large leaf) 3
Roquefort cheese (see Cheese)
Rum (see separate listing, page 102)
Russian dressing (see Salad dressings)
Rutabaga (1 cup cooked) 11.7
Rye bread (see Breads)
Rye whiskey (see separate listing, page 102)
Ry-Krisp (see Crackers)

S

 grams

Salad dressings

Bacon-vinegar (1 tablespoon) 5
Bleu cheese (1 tablespoon) 1.2
Boiled, home-cooked (1 tablespoon) 3.0
Commercial, mayonnaise type (1 tablespoon) ...2.0
French, commercial (1 tablespoon) 3.0
French, homemade (1 tablespoon) 2.0
Italian, commercial (1 tablespoon) 1.0
Mayonnaise (1 tablespoon) 4

Mayonnaise, with mineral oil (1 tablespoon) 1

Roquefort (1 tablespoon) 1.2

Russian (1 tablespoon) 1.5

Thousand Island (1 tablespoon) 2.2

Vinegar and oil, equal parts (1 tablespoon) 4

Salads

Apple-carrot (½ cup) 11.5

Asparagus (5 spears) 3.5

Avocado (½ cup, with dressing) 5.1

Avocado-tomato-cottage cheese 9.3

Banana and nut (½ banana) 15.2

Banana and orange (½ of each) 22.7

Carrot-raisin (3 tablespoons) 27.9

Cole slaw, with French dressing (1 cup) 13.6

Chicken, with celery (½ cup) 2.5

Combination vegetable (½ cup) 15.8

Crab, with celery (½ cup) 3.0

Egg and tomato (1 of each) 4.3

Endive and grapefruit (1 serving) 15.9

Fruit, fresh (3 tablespoons) 21.2

Gelatin, with fruit (1 square) 21.6

Gelatin, with vegetables (1 square) 15.1

Lettuce and tomatoes 5.8

Lettuce with French dressing (1 wedge) 6.9

Lobster, with celery (1 serving) 3.0

Macaroni (1 cup) 48.5

Mixed greens, with French dressing (½ cup) ...4.8

Orange-grapefruit, with dressing 9.5

Potato, with onions (½ cup) 13.1

Prunes, stuffed with cottage cheese (4) 28.2

Salmon, with celery (½ cup) 2.5

Shrimp, with celery (1 serving) 3.0

Tomato and cucumber (1 of each) 8.8

Tomato aspic (½ cup) 5.4

Tuna, with celery (½ cup) 2.5

Waldorf (½ cup) 9.7

Salami (8 ounces) 3.0

Salmon

Broiled or baked 0

Canned 0

Creamed (½ cup, on toast) 16.0

Smoked 0

Salmon loaf (½ cup) 5.1

Salt, table 0

Sand dabs 0

Sandwiches

Bacon-egg (1) 24.5

Bacon-tomato-lettuce (1) 28.8

Barbecue beef (1) 24.0

Barbecue pork (1) 24.0

Bologna (1) 25.6

Cervelat (1) 24.0

Cheese, Camembert (1) 24.4

Cheese, Cheddar (1) 26.4

Cheese, Swiss (1) 24.0
Cheese and olive (1) 25.2
Cheeseburger (1) 22.1
Chicken, sliced (1) 24.0
Chicken liver (1) 25.9
Chicken salad (1) 25.8
Club, 3-decker (1) 41.7
Corned beef (1) 24.0
Crabmeat (1) 25.5
Cream cheese and nut (1) 25.4
Cream cheese and jelly (1) 50.4
Denver, western (1) 27.8
Egg, fried (1) 24.3
Egg salad (1) 24.8
Frankfurter (1) 21.5
Ham, boiled or baked (1) 24.5
Ham, fried (1) 24.0
Ham salad (1) 30.4
Ham and Swiss cheese (1) 25.0
Hamburger (1) 20.9
Liverwurst (1) 24.9
Lobster salad (1) 26.0
Luncheon meat (1) 25.0
Meat loaf (1) 35.9
Oyster, fried (1) 40.7
Pastrami (1) 24.0
Peanut butter (1) 29.3

Peanut butter and jelly (1) 35.3
Pork sausage (1) 24.0
Roast beef (1) 24.0
Roast beef with gravy (1) 27.2
Roast pork (1) 24.0
Roast pork with gravy (1) 27.2
Roquefort spread (1) 25.9
Salami (1) 24.0
Salmon (1) 24.0
Salmon salad (1) 25.2
Sardine (1) 24.0
Shrimp, fried (1, with 6 small) 32.3
Shrimp salad (1) 26.0
Sole, fried (1) 36.0
Steak (1) 24.0
Tomato and lettuce (1) 26.5
Tongue (1) 24.0
Tuna (1) 24.0
Tuna salad (1) 25.8
Turkey (1) 24.0
Turkey with gravy (1) 28.0
Vienna sausage (1) 24.0

Sardines

Canned, in oil 0
Canned, in tomato sauce (1 large) 1.0

Sauces

A-1 (1 tablespoon) 2.7

Barbecue (1 tablespoon) 8.3
Butterscotch (1 tablespoon) 20.2
Caramel (1 tablespoon) 45.8
Cheese (¼ cup) 4.8
Chili (1 tablespoon) 4.0
Cranberry (¼ cup) 35.6
Cream (1 tablespoon) 1.6
Creole (¼ cup) 7.5
Custard (1 tablespoon) 2.3
Fudge (1 tablespoon) 19.0
Garlic, with butter (1 tablespoon) 5
Hard (1 tablespoon) 6.0
Hollandaise, mock (¼ cup) 6.3
Hollandaise, true (¼ cup) 4
Lemon (1 tablespoon) 6.9
Marshmallow (1 tablespoon) 6.2
Meat, Italian (1 cup) 20.8
Mustard (¼ cup) 6.4
Raisin (¼ cup) 25.9
Sour cream (1 tablespoon) 3.5
Soy (1 tablespoon) 1.5
Tartar (1 tablespoon) 1.5
Tomato (¼ cup) 6.0
White, medium (¼ cup) 6.1
White, thin (¼ cup) 4.6
Worcestershire (1 tablespoon) 2.7

Sauerkraut (1 cup drained) 7.0
Sauerkraut juice (see Juices)
Sausage, bologna (see Bologna)
Sausage, cervelat (see Cervelat)
Sausage, frankfurter (see Frankfurter)
Sausage, liver (see Liverwurst)
Sausage, Polish (4 ounces) 1.3
Sausage, pork (8 ounces) ....trace
Sausage, salami (see Salami)
Sausage, Vienna, canned (8 ounces) 7
Scallions (see Onions, green)
Scallops (2-3) 3.4
Scallops, fried with batter (3-4 large) 14.6
Scampi (see Shrimp)
Scotch whisky (see separate listing, page 102)
Scrapple (1 medium slice) 26.0
Seafood (see individual listings)
Seafood au gratin (½ cup) 12.1
Seltzer water (see Soft drinks, soda)
Sesame seeds (1 ounce) .... trace
Shad 0
Sherbets (see Ice cream, ices)
Sherry (see separate listing, page 103)
Shortbread (see Breads)
Shortcake, peach (small serving) 42.4
Shortcake, raspberry (medium serving) 47.4
Shortcake, strawberry (medium serving) 61.2

Shortcake, strawberry sponge (medium serving) 60.4
Shortening (see Butter, Crisco, or Lard)
Shredded wheat (see Cereals)
Shrimp
    Fresh (7 large or 8 ounces) 2.4
    Canned, dry pack (3 ounces) 8
    Canned, wet pack (3 ounces) 4
    Fried, with batter (3 jumbo) 8.3
    Scampi (7 large, in garlic butter) 3.6
Shrimp cocktail (with sauce) 4.8
Shrimp creole (7 large with ½ cup sauce) 17.4
Smelt 0
Smelt, fried with batter (2-3) .10.8
Snap beans (see Beans, green and wax)
Snow peas (14-16) 5.6
Sodas (see Soft drinks or Ice cream sodas)
Sole 0
Soft drinks
    Cherry (8 ounces) 28.0
    Coca Cola (8 ounces) 27.0
    Cream soda (8 ounces) .28.0
    Ginger ale (8 ounces) 21.0
    Grape (8 ounces) 28.0
    Lemon (8 ounces) 28.0
    Low calorie, most flavors (8 ounces) 0
    Orange (8 ounces) 28.0
    Pepsi Cola (8 ounces) 27.0

Root beer (8 ounces) 28.0

Sarsaparilla (8 ounces) 28.0

Soda, seltzer water (8 ounces) 0

Quinine water (8 ounces) 9.0

Soups (each serving approximately ¾ cup)

Asparagus, cream (1 serving) 12.5

Bean (1 serving) 18.5

Beef noodle (1 serving) 4.6

Beef with vegetable and barley (1 serving) 7.0

Bouillon (1 serving) 0

Celery, cream (1 serving) 12.0

Chicken broth (1 serving) 0

Chicken, cream (1 serving) 11.8

Chicken, gumbo (1 serving) 12.4

Chicken, noodle (1 serving) 6.5

Chicken, rice (1 serving) 4.6

Chicken vegetable (1 serving) 7.0

Chili beef (1 serving) 18.9

Clam chowder, milk (1 serving) 13.5

Clam chowder, tomato (1 serving) 8.3

Consommé (1 serving) 0

Corn chowder (1 serving) 19.0

Green pea (1 serving) 17.5

Green pea with ham (1 serving) 14.6

Gumbo creole (1 serving) 9.5

Jellied consommé (1 serving) 0

Mushroom, cream (1 serving) 13.2

Noodle (1 serving) 6.9
Onion (1 serving) 3.9
Onion, cream (1 serving) 6.8
Onion, French (1 serving) 3.9
Oyster stew (see Oysters)
Pea, cream (1 serving) 22.6
Pepperpot (1 serving) 8.0
Potato, cream (1 serving) 13.8
Scotch broth (1 serving) 9.1
Shrimp, cream (1 serving) 12.0
Spinach, cream (1 serving) 11.1
Split pea (1 serving) 16.9
Tomato, clear (1 serving) 12.0
Tomato, cream (1 serving) 14.5
Tomato rice (1 serving) 12.7
Tomato vegetable (1 serving) 11.0
Turkey noodle (1 serving) 7.0
Turtle (1 serving) 7.0
Vegetable (1 serving) 10.5
Vegetable, beef (1 serving) 7.1
Vegetable, cream (1 serving) 9.9
Vichyssoise (1 serving) 12.2
Soybean curd (1 cake) 3.0
Soybean milk (⅜ cup) 2.1
Soybean sprouts (1 cup) 10.8
Soybeans (see Beans)
Spaghetti

Cooked (1 cup) 44.1
Cooked, with meat sauce (1 serving) 39.4
Cooked, with meatballs (¾ cup, 6 meatballs) ...43.6
Cooked, with tomato sauce (1 serving) 34.3
Spareribs (see Pork)
Spices (1 teaspoon) 0
Spinach
    Raw (½ pound) 5.9
    Cooked (1 cup) 7.2
    Canned (1 cup, drained) 6.4
    Canned, strained, creamed (1 ounce) 2.0
Split pea soup (see Soups)
Spoon bread (see Breads)
Squab 0
Squash
    Hubbard or winter, baked (½ cup) 15.0
    Hubbard or winter, frozen, boiled (1 cup) 9.7
    Summer, boiled (1 cup drained) 7.0
    Summer, canned, strained (1 ounce) 1.4
    Zucchini, boiled (1 cup drained) 6.3
Squid 0
Stew
    Beef and vegetable (1 cup) 17.0
    Lamb and vegetable (1 cup) 11.3
    Oyster (see Oysters)
    Rabbit (1 cup) 11.3
    Veal and vegetables (1 cup) 11.3

Strawberries

    Fresh (5 large) 4.2

    Fresh (1 cup) 13.0

    Frozen (10-ounce carton) 75.0

    Frozen (16-ounce can) 100.0

String beans (see Beans, green)

Stroganoff (medium serving) 7.0

Stuffing, bread (½ cup) 28.5

Sturgeon 0

Succotash, canned (½ cup) 17.6

Succotash, frozen (½ cup) 18.9

Sugar

    Beet (¼ pound) 112.7

    Brown (1 cup) 210.0

    Brown (1 tablespoon) 13.0

    Confectioner's (1 cup) 127.4

    Confectioner's (1 tablespoon) 8.0

    Granulated (1 cup) 199.0

    Granulated (1 tablespoon) 12.0

    Granulated (1 teaspoon) 4.0

    Granulated (3 cubes) 7.0

    Granulated (1 lump) 7.0

    Maple (1-inch cube) 27.0

Sugar cane juice (5 tablespoons) 72.6

Summer squash (see Squash)

Sundaes (see Ice cream sundaes)

Sweet potatoes (see Potatoes, sweet)

Sweetbreads 0

Sweetbreads, creamed (½ cup) 6.1

Swiss chard (see Chard)

Swordfish 0

Syrups

    Chocolate thin-type (1 tablespoon) 12.0

    Chocolate, fudge-type (1 tablespoon) 10.5

    Corn (1 cup) 242.0

    Corn (1 tablespoon) 15.0

    Corn (1 plastic packet) 37.0

    Honey (1 tablespoon) 16.4

    Maple (1 tablespoon) 12.8

    Molasses, light (1 tablespoon) 13.0

    Molasses, medium (1 tablespoon) 12.0

    Molasses, blackstrap (1 tablespoon) 11.0

    Molasses, Barbados (1 tablespoon) 14.0

    Simple sugar (1 tablespoon) 7.0

    Sorghum (3 ounces) 13.4

    Treacle (1 tablespoon) 13.4

grams

Tangerine juice (see Juices)

Tangerines (1 medium) 10.0

Tapioca (¼ cup dry) 32.8

Tapioca pudding (see Puddings)

Taro, Hawaiian, tubers (3½ ounces) 25.0

Taro, Japanese, Dasheen (3½ ounces) 21.2

Taro, leaves and stems (3½ ounces) 21.2

Tea (1 cup) 4

Tea, with 1 tbs. light cream 9

Tea, with 1 tbs. heavy cream 8

Tea, with 1 teaspoon lemon 8

Tea, with 1 tablespoon milk 1.1

Tea, with 1 teaspoon sugar 4.4

Thousand Island dressing (see Salad dressings)

Toast, bread (see Breads, carbohydrate value unchanged)

Toast, Holland rusk (1) 8.6

Toast, Melba (1 slice) 3.9

Toast, zwieback (1 slice) 5.1

Tomato catsup (see Catsup)

Tomato juice (see Juices)

Tomato sauce (see Sauces)

Tomato soup (see Soups)

Tomatoes

    Fresh (1 medium) 6.0

    Fresh (1 small) 4.0

    Canned (1 cup) 9.0

    Purée, canned (1 cup) 18.0

    Stewed (1 cup) 9.0

Tongue, beef (see Beef)

Tongue, canned (3 medium slices) 2

Tortilla (1 5-inch) 4.5

Tripe, boiled 0

Tripe, pickled 0

Trout, brook 0

Trout, lake 0

Tuna

    Fresh or canned 0

    Casserole, with noodles (1 serving) 25.0

Turkey

    Roasted or smoked 0

    Creamed (4 ounces) 6.1

    Pot pie, frozen (8 ounces) 50.4

    Potted 0

Turkey hash (see Hash)

Turnip greens (1 cup cooked) 8.0

Turnip greens, canned (1 cup) 7.0

Turnips (1 cup diced) 9.0

Turnips, cooked (1) 4.7
Turtle 0

                           grams

Vanilla extract (1 teaspoon) 1
Vanilla ice cream (see Ice cream)
Vanilla pudding (see Puddings)
Veal
    Chop 0
    Cutlet 0
    Cutlet, breaded (1 medium) 16.0
    Kidney (see Kidneys)
    Roast 0
    Stew (see Stew)
    Stewing meat 0
Veal goulash (see Goulash, Hungarian)
Vegetable juice (see Juices)
Vegetable and meat stew (see Stew)
Vegetable soup (see Soups)
Vegetables (see individual listings)
Vegetables, mixed, canned (4 ounces) 15.1

Vegetables, mixed, frozen (4 ounces) 15.7
Venison 0
Vienna sausage (see Sausage)
Vinegar (1 tablespoon) 8

                                                    grams

Waffles (1 medium) 30.0
Walnuts, black (1 cup chopped) 19.0
Walnuts, black (8 to 10 halves) 2.8
Walnuts, English (8 to 16 halves) 2.3
Walnuts, English (1 cup chopped) 17.6
Walnuts, English (1 tablespoon chopped) 1.0
Water chestnuts (4) 4.5
Water cress (see Cress)
Watermelon (1 slice, 1½" x 6") 38.4
Watermelon (1 wedge, 1/16 of melon) 57.6
Watermelon, balls or cubes (½ cup) 6.9
Wax beans (see Beans)
Welsh rabbit (medium serving, on toast) 23.5
Wheat germ (1 tablespoon) 3.7
Whipped cream (see Cream)

White fish, steamed or smoked 0
White fish, baked, stuffed (1 serving) 11.6
White sauce (see Sauces)
Wine (see separate listing, page 103)

.grams

Yams (see Potatoes, sweet)
Yeast (1 cake) 3.7
Yeast, dried (1 tablespoon) 3.0
Yogurt, skim milk (1 cup) 11.7

Zucchini (see Squash)
Zwiebach (see Toast)

ALCOHOLIC BEVERAGES

.grams

Beers, ciders
    Ale, light (8 ounces) 8.0
    Ale, imported (8 ounces) 10.0
    Beer (8 ounces) 11.0
    Cider, fermented (6 ounces) 1.8
    Porter or stout (8 ounces) 10.0
Cocktails, highballs
    Alexander, brandy (1) 4.0
    Bacardi cocktail (1) 3.3
    Bloody Mary (1) 5.1
    Bourbon highball, soda (1) 0
    Bourbon highball, ginger ale 15.7
    Champagne cocktail (1) 9.0
    Daiquiri (1) 5.2
    Eggnog (1) 18.0
    Gimlet (1) 1.2
    Gin and tonic (10 ounces) 9.0
    Gin rickey (1) 1.3
    Grasshopper (1) 18.0
    Hot buttered rum (1) ....trace
    Irish coffee (1) 5.5
    Manhattan (1) 7.9
    Martini (1) 3
    Mint julep (1) 2.7
    Old fashioned (1) 3.5
    Orange blossom (1) 3.7

Pink lady (1) 3.0

Planter's punch (1) 7.9

Rob Roy, with dry vermouth (1) 1

Rum and cola (1) 20.4

Rum punch (1) 7.9

Rye highball, ginger ale (1) 15.7

Rye highball, soda (1) 0

Sazarac (1) 2.5

Scotch highball, soda (1) 0

Scotch mist (1) 0

Screwdriver (1) 15.0

Sidecar (1) 4.2

Sloe gin fizz (1) 1.3

Stinger (1) 9.0

Tom Collins (1) 9.0

Whiskey sour (1) 3.9

Liquors, whiskeys

Bourbon whiskey (1½ ounces) 0

Canadian whiskey (1½ ounces) 0

Gin (1½ ounces) 0

Irish whiskey (1½ ounces) 0

Rum (1½ ounces) 0

Rye whiskey (1½ ounces) 0

Scotch whisky (1½ ounces) 0

Sloe gin (1½ ounces) 0

Vodka (1½ ounces) 0

Liqueurs, brandies

Anisette (1 ounce) 7.0

Applejack (1 ounce) ....trace
Benedictine (1 ounce) 6.6
Brandy (1 ounce) 0
Chartreuse (1 ounce) 6.6
Cherry Heering (1 ounce) 6.0
Crème de cacao (1 ounce) 6.0
Crème de menthe (1 ounce) 6.0
Curaçao (1 ounce) 6.0
Kummel (1 ounce) 6.0

Wines

Champagne, dry, domestic (4 ounces) 3.0
Champagne, dry, French (4 ounces) 1.0
Dinner, dry red—Chianti, Claret,
    Burgundy (3½ ounces) 5
Dinner, dry white—Chablis, Moselle,
Rhine (3½ ounces) 5
Dinner, white—Sauterne (3½ ounces) 4.0
Dubonnet (3 ounces) 12.0
Madeira (3½ ounces) 3.0
Malaga (3½ ounces) 20.0
Muscatel (3½ ounces) 14.0
Port (3½ ounces) 14.0
Sherry (3½ ounces) 4.8
Vermouth, dry (3½ ounces) 1.0
Vermouth, sweet (3½ ounces) 12.0

LOW-GRAM SNACKS & TIDBITS

	grams
Almonds, salted (12–15)	2.9
Anchovy fillets (8)	trace
Anchovy paste (1 teaspoon)	.3
Bacon (2 strips)	.2
Brazil nuts, in shell (10)	4.8
Capers (1 tablespoon)	trace
Carrot sticks, raw (3)	2.8
Cashew nuts (6 to 8)	4.1
Caviar (1 ounce)	1.1
Celery (1 large stalk)	1.5

Cheese

	grams
American (1 ounce)	.6
Bleu (1 ounce)	.6
Brie (1 ounce)	.5
Camembert (1 ounce)	.5
Chateau (1 ounce)	1.1
Cheddar (1 ounce)	.6
Cream (1 tablespoon)	.3
Edam (1 ounce)	1.1
Gruyere (1 ounce)	.5
Liederkranz (1 ounce)	.6
Limburger (1 ounce)	.6
Swiss (1 ounce)	.5

	grams
Cheese spreads, bleu, bacon, olive, etc. (1 ounce)	1.9
Chicken, canned, boned	.0
Clams, cherrystone or littleneck (6)	4.5
Clams, canned, drained (3 ounces)	1.6

Crab paste (1 teaspoon) 1

Crab salad (½ cup) 3.0

Crackers

    Cheese tidbits (15 tiny) 3.0

    Rye thin (1) 1.9

    Wheat thin (1) 1.3

Dip, onion with sour cream (1 tablespoon) 1.5

Dip, seafood with sour cream (1 tablespoon) 4

Eel, smoked 0

Eggs, deviled (1) 5

Egg roll (1) 3.5

Filberts (10 to 12) 2.6

Frankfurter (1 cooked, about 1.8 ounces) 1.0

Frankfurter, cocktail (1, 2-inches long) 4

Gefilte fish (2 ounces) 4.8

Gum, chewing (1 stick) 1.7

Gum, candy coated (1 piece) 1.3

Ham, boiled or prosciutto 0

Hazelnuts (10–12) 3.0

Herring, raw, pickled or smoked 0

Herring, marinated with sour cream (1 small piece) .8

Hickory nuts (15 small) 2.0

Liver, chicken, chopped (3 ounces) 3.0

Liver spread (2 tablespoons) 2

Lobster cocktail (½ cup meat, 1 tbs. mayonnaise) .. .9

Lobster paste (1 teaspoon) 1

Meatballs, cocktail (all meat) 0

Mints, after-dinner (5 small) 1.3

Mussels, smoked (1) .... trace

Nuts, mixed (8 to 12) 2.7

Olives, green (5 large) 5
Olives, black (5 large) 1.0
Oysters, raw (3 to 4 medium) 4.0
Oysters, smoked (4 to 6 small) 2.6
Pâté de foie gras (1 tablespoon) 7
Pecans (12 nutmeats) 1.8
Peanuts (10) 2.1
Pepper, green (½ medium) 1.5
Pickle, dill (½ large) 1.5
Pickle, sour (½ large) 1.5
Pickle, sweet gherkin (1 medium) 2.6
Pig's feet 0
Pistachio nuts (20) 1.6
Polish sausage (4 ounces) 1.3
Pork sausage (8 ounces) ....trace
Pretzels (5 sticks) 1.4
Salmon, canned 0
Salmon salad (½ cup) 2.5
Sardines, canned in oil 0
Shrimp (7 large) 2.4
Tuna, canned 0
Tunafish salad (½ cup) 2.5
Tripe, pickled 0
Vienna sausage, canned (3 pieces) ....trace
Walnuts, English (8-16 halves) 2.3

TWO WEEKS OF LOW-GRAM MENUS

The fourteen menus that follow are typical low-gram meals—tempting and tantalizing, but still within the 60 grams a day you're allowed on this dream of a diet. Bear in mind, however, that these menus are merely suggestions, and you are, of course, free to make substitutions as you please. Simply be accurate about substitutions—and, especially if you're going to stay on the diet longer than two weeks, pick foods that have the same, or similar, nutritional value.

You'll notice as you glance at the menus that some foods are listed by specific amount and/or weight (for example, "2 eggs," "2 tbs. sour cream," "1 cup cabbage") and other foods are listed only by name (for example, "sirloin steak," "roast duck," "ground round"). The difference in the two kinds of listings is simple: when a specific amount is called for, it means that the dedicated dieter should eat <u>exactly</u> that amount, <u>period</u>; when no amount is specified, it means the dieter may eat as much of the food as he wishes. That's the beauty of the low-carbohydrate diet. You don't ever have to feign contentment or pretend fulfillment. Still hungry after you've eaten everything on the menu? Don't hold back. Have another hamburger, a third lamb chop, a turkey leg! Chances are, you won't be hungry on this diet, but if you are, there's no need to <u>stay</u> hungry, no need to suffer, no need to get tense and irritable. Try it. You'll see. You have nothing to lose but those extra pounds.

DAY 1

BREAKFAST	grams
2 eggs, fried	.6
in 2 tbs. butter	.2
4 bacon strips	.4
½ hamburger roll, toasted,	10.5
spread with 1 tbs. butter	.1
1 cup coffee with 1 tbs. heavy cream	1.2
	13.0

LUNCH	
1 rye, Scotch or bourbon highball (water or soda)	.0
½ medium California avocado,	6.0
topped with 3 tbs. oil and vinegar (equal parts)	1.2
6 oz. cured baked ham slices	.6
2 oz. Swiss cheese slices	1.0
1 slice Holland rusk toast	8.6
1 cup coffee with 1 tbs. heavy cream	1.2
	18.6

DINNER	
1 gin or vodka martini	.3
8 small anchovy fillets	trace
and 1 medium canned pimiento,	2.2
sprinkled with 1 tsp. lemon juice	.4
sirloin steak	.0
½ cup mashed (with milk and butter) potatoes	14.0
10 inner leaves endive,	1.0
topped with 2 tbs. bacon-vinegar dressing	1.0
1 glass (3½ oz.) dry red wine	.5
1 oz. Liederkranz cheese	.6
2 rye thins	3.8
total for the day: 55.4+	23.8

DAY 2

BREAKFAST grams

2 eggs, scrambled, ...6
    with smoked salmon slices, diced, ...0
    and 2 tbs. chopped onions 2.0
    in 2 tbs. butter 2
½ slice white bread, toasted, ... 6.0
    spread with 1 tbs. butter 1
1 cup coffee with 1 tbs. heavy cream 1.2

                                        10.1

LUNCH

1 Rob Roy (with dry vermouth) 1
½ cup melon balls, frozen 6.3
1 cup canned lamb or veal and vegetable stew 11.3
¾ cup shredded cabbage 4.0
    and ½ medium green pepper, diced, ... 1.5
    topped with 2 tbs. mayonnaise 8
1 cup iced coffee, topped with 2 tbs. whipped cream 1.2

                                        25.2

DINNER

½ medium tomato 3.0
    stuffed with ¼ cup crabmeat salad 1.5
short ribs of beef, ...0
    braised with 3½ oz. dry red wine 5
½ cup cooked fresh green beans, ... 3.0
    topped with 2 tbs. butter 2
10 small leaves iceberg lettuce, ... 2.5
    topped with 2 tbs. Roquefort dressing 2.4
10 large fresh cherries 10.0
1 oz. brandy 0

total for the day: 58.4   23.1

DAY 3

BREAKFAST	grams
½ cup tomato juice	5.2
2 eggs, poached, ...	.6
on 1 slice white bread, toasted, ...	11.9
spread with 1 tbs. butter	.1
3 bacon slices	.3
1 cup coffee with 1 tbs. heavy cream	1.2
	19.3

LUNCH	
1 gin or vodka martini	.3
chopped sirloin steak or ground round	.0
½ cup cooked fresh broccoli, ...	4.1
topped with 2 tbs. melted butter	.2
tomato-cucumber (½ of each) salad, ...	4.4
topped with 2 tbs. Italian dressing	2.0
1 cup coffee with 1 tbs. heavy cream	1.2
	12.2

DINNER	
¾ cup French onion soup, ...	3.9
with 1 tsp. grated Parmesan cheese	.1
roast duck	.0
½ cup wild rice	15.1
6 cooked fresh asparagus stalks	3.0
topped with 3 tbs. Hollandaise sauce	.3
1 glass (3½ oz.) dry white wine	.5
1 ounce Brie cheese	.5
with 2 rye thins	3.8
1 cup coffee with 1 oz. Irish whiskey	.8
and 1 tbs. whipped cream	.2
total for the day: 59.7	28.2

DAY 4

BREAKFAST grams

½ cup fresh strawberries, ... 6.5
    topped with 3 tbs. heavy cream 1.2
2 eggs, scrambled, ...6
    in 2 tbs. butter 2
4 pork sausages ....trace
1 cup coffee with 1 tbs. heavy cream 1.2
                                             9.7

LUNCH

1 rye, Scotch or bourbon highball (water or soda) .0
3 oz. chopped chicken liver, ... 3.0
    sprinkled with 1 tsp. lemon juice 4
lamb chops 0
6 large fresh mushrooms, ... 6.0
    sautéed in 2 tbs. butter 2
½ cup mixed green salad, ... 2.0
    topped with 2 tbs. Russian dressing 3.0
1 cup iced tea with 1 tsp. lemon juice 8
                                           15.4

DINNER

7 large fresh shrimp (8 oz.), ... 2.4
    cooked in 2 tbs. garlic butter 2
prime ribs of beef 0
½ baked potato, ...10.5
    topped with 2 tbs. sour cream and chopped
        chives 1.0
½ cup cooked fresh spinach 3.6
1 glass (3½ oz.) dry red wine 5
1 slice gold cake 14.8
1 cup coffee with 1 tbs. heavy cream 1.2
total for the day: 59.3   34.2

DAY 5

BREAKFAST	grams
½ cup vegetable juice	4.3
cheese omelette (with 2 eggs)	.9
3 Canadian bacon slices	.2
2 rye thins, ...	3.8
spread with 1 tbs. butter	.1
and 1 tsp. strawberry jam	4.8
1 cup coffee with 1 tbs. heavy cream	1.2
	15.3

LUNCH

	grams
1 Rob Roy (with dry vermouth)	.1
1 cup jellied consommé	.0
hot turkey slices	.0
with 4 tbs. cranberries	3.0
1 medium cucumber, sliced, ...	2.8
and ¼ small tomato, sliced, ...	1.0
topped with 2 tbs. mayonnaise	.8
½ cup fresh orange sections, ...	11.0
topped with 4 tbs. dry red wine	.3
	19.0

DINNER

	grams
Italian antipasto (5 large black olives, 4 anchovy fillets, proscuitto ham, 1 medium pimiento, 1 oz. provolone cheese, sardines)	4.0
veal cutlets, ...	.0
topped with ¼ cup tomato sauce	6.0
and 3 oz. grated Parmesan cheese	2.4
½ cup cooked fresh Brussels sprouts	6.2
1 glass (3½ oz.) dry white wine	.5
1 cup espresso with 1 tbs. whipped cream	1.0
total for the day: 54.4	20.1

DAY 6

BREAKFAST	grams
¼ cantaloupe melon	4.2
sturgeon slices	.0
and 2 tbs. cream cheese,	.6
atop 3 pieces Melba toast	11.7
1 cup coffee with 1 tbs. heavy cream	1.2
	17.7

LUNCH

	grams
1 gin or vodka martini	.3
1 cup clear chicken broth	.0
1 medium green pepper, halved,	3.0
stuffed with ground beef	.0
1 cup shredded cabbage,	5.4
topped with 2 tbs. mayonnaise	.8
and 1 tsp. lemon juice	.4
1 medium fresh peach, sliced,	9.7
topped with 2 tbs. sour cream	1.0
	20.6

DINNER

	grams
1 wedge honeydew melon	12.8
with proscuitto ham slices	.0
roast pork	.0
6 cooked fresh asparagus stalks,	3.0
topped with 2 tbs. cheese sauce	2.4
7 small leaves escarole	.8
and 4 anchovy fillets, diced,	trace
topped with 1 tbs. Roquefort dressing	1.2
1 cup espresso with 1 tbs. heavy cream	1.0
1 oz. brandy	.0
total for the day: 59.5	21.2

DAY 7

BREAKFAST grams

½ cup fresh black raspberries, ...10.5
    with 1 tsp. confectioner's sugar 2.7
    and ¼ cup light cream 2.1
2 eggs, fried 6
    in 2 tbs. butter 2
2 rye thins, ... 3.8
    spread with 1 tbs. cream cheese 3
1 cup coffee with 1 tbs. heavy cream 1.2

21.4

LUNCH

1 rye, Scotch or bourbon highball (water or soda) .. .0
flank steak or London broil slices 0
4 large fresh mushrooms, ... 4.0
    sautéed in 3 tbs. butter 3
½ cup cooked fresh broccoli 4.1
½ cup watermelon balls, ... 6.9
    topped with 4 tbs. dry red wine 3

15.6

DINNER

1 gin or vodka martini 3
7 large fresh shrimp (8 oz.) 2.4
    with 2 tbs. mayonnaise 8
African lobster tails 0
    with ¼ cup melted butter 4
6–8 potato chips 8.0
½ cup cole slaw 6.8
1 glass (3½ oz.) dry white wine 5
1 cup coffee with 1 tbs. heavy cream 1.2
total for the day: 57.4 20.4

DAY 8

BREAKFAST	grams
½ cup puffed rice	5.8
with ¼ cup light cream	2.1
and 3 tbs. fresh blueberries	4.0
2 eggs, soft-boiled	.6
1 cup coffee with 1 tbs. heavy cream	1.2
	13.7

LUNCH	
¼ cantaloupe melon	4.2
2 frankfurters,	2.0
with 1 tbs. prepared mustard	.8
½ cup sauerkraut	3.5
sprinkled with ½ tsp. fresh chopped dill	.0
6 oz. light ale	6.0
1 medium sour pickle	2.5
	19.0

DINNER	
2 large stalks celery,	3.0
stuffed with 1 oz. Roquefort cheese	.5
mixed with 1 oz. cream cheese	.6
roast chicken	.0
½ cup creamed potatoes	14.1
½ small tomato, broiled	2.0
½ cup cooked green beans,	3.0
topped with 2 tbs. butter	.2
and 4 chopped salted almonds	1.0
1 oz. Brie cheese	.5
1 cup coffee with 1 oz. Irish whiskey	.8
and 1 tbs. whipped cream	.2
total for the day: 58.6	25.9

DAY 9

BREAKFAST	grams
½ cup tomato juice	5.2
2 eggs, scrambled, ...	.6
in 2 tbs. butter	.2
smelt, fried	.0
in 4 tbs. butter	.4
1 cup coffee with 1 tbs. heavy cream	1.2
	7.6

LUNCH	
1 Rob Roy (with dry vermouth)	.1
chopped sirloin steak or ground round, ...	.0
atop ½ hamburger roll, toasted, ...	10.5
sprinkled with 1 tbs. chopped onion	1.0
6 small leaves iceberg lettuce	1.5
and ¼ medium tomato, sliced, ...	1.5
and ½ medium green pepper, sliced, ...	1.5
topped with 2 tbs. Thousand Island dressing ..	4.4
1 cup iced coffee with 1 tbs. heavy cream	1.2
	21.7

DINNER	
1 old-fashioned	3.5
2 Ritz crackers	4.2
spread with 1 tsp. anchovy paste and 1 tsp. butter	.3
pork chops	.0
2 tbs. canned unsweetened applesauce	3.3
½ cup cooked fresh carrots, diced	4.7
½ cup cooked cauliflower	3.0
10 fresh large strawberries, ...	8.4
topped with 4 tbs. dry red wine	.3
total for the day: 57.0	27.7

DAY 10

BREAKFAST grams

2-egg plain omelette, cooked in 2 tbs. butter	.8
½ hamburger roll, toasted,	10.5
spread with 1 tbs. butter	.1
3 strips bacon	.3
1 cup coffee with 1 tbs. heavy cream	1.2
	12.9

LUNCH

1 gin or vodka martini	.3
3 pieces herring, marinated in sour cream	2.4
cold corned beef slices,	.0
topped with 1 tbs. Russian dressing,	1.5
on 1 slice light rye bread	12.1
4 large green olives	.4
4 pieces chowchow pickles	1.1
6 tbs. potato salad	9.0
1 cup iced tea with 1 tsp. lemon	.8
	27.6

DINNER

1 rye, Scotch or bourbon highball (water or soda)	3.0
¾ cup French onion soup,	3.9
sprinkled with 2 tsp. grated Parmesan cheese	.1
roast leg of lamb	.0
½ cup cubed California avocado,	4.5
topped with 2 tbs. vinegar and oil (equal parts)	.8
6 cooked fresh asparagus stalks,	3.0
topped with 4 tbs. Hollandaise sauce	.4
1 cup coffee with 1 oz. Irish whiskey	.8
and 1 tbs. whipped cream	.2
total for the day: 57.2	16.7

DAY 11

BREAKFAST grams
½ cup fresh grapefruit sections 9.8
2 eggs, soft boiled 6
3 oz. baked ham slices 3
1 saltine, ... 2.9
    spread with 1 tbs. butter 1
1 cup coffee with 1 tbs. heavy cream 1.2
                                       14.9

LUNCH
1 cup jellied consommé, ...0
    sprinkled with 1 tsp. chopped chives 0
12 clams, steamed 8.6
    with 4 tbs. butter 4
½ cup shredded cabbage, ... 2.7
    topped with 2 tbs. mayonnaise 8
1 glass (3½ oz.) dry white wine 5
1 oz. Camembert cheese 5
2 rye thins 3.8
                                       17.3

DINNER
1 whiskey sour 3.9
4–6 small smoked oysters 2.6
porterhouse steak 0
½ baked potato, ...10.5
    topped with 2 tbs. sour cream and
        chopped chives 1.0
10 inner leaves endive 1.0
    topped with 2 tbs. bacon-vinegar dressing ... 1.0
½ cup cooked fresh spinach 3.6
1 cup coffee with 1 tbs. heavy cream 1.2
total for the day: 57.0   24.8

DAY 12

BREAKFAST grams

2 eggs, poached, ...6
   atop 1 slice white bread, toasted, ...11.9
     spread with 1 tbs. butter 1
4 pork sausages ....trace
1 cup coffee with 1 tbs. heavy cream 1.2
                                              13.8

LUNCH

1 rye, Scotch or bourbon highball (water or soda).. .0
¾ cup beef noodle soup 4.6
cold roast beef slices 0
cold turkey or chicken slices 0
2 oz. Gruyere cheese 1.0
½ cup Waldorf salad 9.7
1 cup tea with 1 tsp. lemon juice 8
2 sugar-wafer cookies 3.0
                                            19.1

DINNER

1 gin or vodka martini 3
4 Ritz crackers, spread with 8.4
   1 tbs. caviar (red or black) 5
   mixed with 1 tbs. sour cream 5
lake or brook trout, ...0
   basted with 2 tbs. butter, ...2
   topped with 6 chopped salted almonds 1.5
½ cup cooked fresh green beans 3.0
½ cup stewed tomatoes 4.5
1 cup espresso with 1 tbs. whipped cream 1.0
1 oz. brandy 0
total for the day: 52.8+   19.9

DAY 13

BREAKFAST   grams
½ cup fresh peach slices 8.0
smoked salmon slices 0
smoked white fish slices 0
½ slice light rye bread, toasted, ... 6.1
    spread with 1 tbs. cream cheese 3
1 cup coffee with 1 tbs. heavy cream 1.2
                                               15.6

LUNCH
½ medium green pepper, ... 1.5
    stuffed with 1 cup chicken salad 4.8
½ medium tomato, broiled 3.0
    with 1 tsp. grated Parmesan cheese 1
1 slice zwiebach toast 5.1
    spread with 1 tbs. butter 1
1 glass (3½ oz.) dry white wine 5
½ slice pound cake, ... 7.4
    topped with 5 fresh large strawberries 4.2
                                               26.7

DINNER
1 rye, Scotch or bourbon highball (water or soda) .. .0
1 cup chicken broth 0
2 large stalks celery 3.0
    with 2 tbs. onion dip (with sour cream) 3.0
flank steak or London broil slices 0
10 small leaves iceberg lettuce, ... 2.5
    topped with 1 tbs. Roquefort cheese dressing . 1.2
½ cup boiled summer squash 3.5
1 cup coffee with Irish whiskey 8
total for the day: 56.3   14.0

DAY 14

BREAKFAST   grams
½ cup vegetable juice 4.3
2 eggs, scrambled, ...6
    in 2 tbs. butter 2
½ hamburger roll, toasted, ...10.5
    spread with 1 tbs. butter 1
3 Canadian bacon slices 2
1 cup coffee with 1 tbs. heavy cream 1.2
                                                              17.1

LUNCH
1 gin or vodka martini 3
4 cherrystone or littleneck clams 3.0
    with 1 tsp. catsup 1.4
    and 2 tsp. lemon juice 8
swordfish steak 0
    basted with 2 tbs. butter and 1 tsp.
        anchovy paste 5
3 canned artichoke hearts 5.0
    with 2 tbs. Hollandaise sauce 2
1 cup tea with lemon 8
                                                              12.0

DINNER
¾ cup cream of onion soup 6.8
2 rye thins 3.8
    spread with 1 tbs. Old English cheese spread 1.0
fried chicken (½ bird dipped in flour) 6.2
½ cup cooked fresh beets 8.1
1 medium cucumber, sliced, ... 2.8
    topped with 2 tbs. sour cream and
        chopped chives 1.0
1 glass (3½ oz.) white wine 5
total for the day: 59.3   30.2

TOTAL YOUR GRAMS

DAY 1:
    breakfast ....
    lunch ....
    dinner ....
    snacks ....
                         daily total:

DAY 2:
    breakfast ....
    lunch ....
    dinner ....
    snacks ....
                         daily total:

DAY 3:
    breakfast ....
    lunch ....
    dinner ....
    snacks ....
                         daily total:

DAY 4:
    breakfast ....
    lunch ....
    dinner ....
    snacks ....
                         daily total:

DAY 5:
    breakfast ....
    lunch ....
    dinner ....
    snacks ....
                         daily total:

DAY 6:
    breakfast ....
    lunch ....
    dinner ....
    snacks ....
                   daily total:

DAY 7:
    breakfast ....
    lunch ....
    dinner ....
    snacks ....
                   daily total:

DAY 8:
    breakfast ....
    lunch ....
    dinner ....
    snacks ....
                   daily total:

DAY 9:
    breakfast ....
    lunch ....
    dinner ....
    snacks ....
                   daily total:

DAY 10:
    breakfast ....
    lunch ....
    dinner ....
    snacks ....
                   daily total:

DAY 11:
    breakfast ....
    lunch ....
    dinner ....
    snacks ....
                  daily total:

DAY 12:
    breakfast ....
    lunch ....
    dinner ....
    snacks ....
                  daily total:

DAY 13:
    breakfast ....
    lunch ....
    dinner ....
    snacks ....
                  daily total:

DAY 14:
    breakfast ....
    lunch ....
    dinner ....
    snacks ....
                  daily total:

WHAT YOU SHOULD WEIGH   WOMEN

height*	small frame	medium frame	large frame
4 ft. 10 in.	92-98	96-107	104-119
4 ft. 11 in.	94-101	98-110	106-122
5 ft. 0 in.	96-104	101-113	109-125
5 ft. 1 in.	99-107	104-116	112-128
5 ft. 2 in.	102-110	107-119	115-131
5 ft. 3 in.	105-113	110-122	118-134
5 ft. 4 in.	108-116	113-126	121-138
5 ft. 5 in.	111-119	116-130	125-142
5 ft. 6 in.	114-123	120-135	129-146
5 ft. 7 in.	118-127	124-139	133-150
5 ft. 8 in.	122-131	128-143	137-154
5 ft. 9 in.	126-135	132-147	141-158
5 ft. 10 in.	130-140	136-151	145-163
5 ft. 11 in.	134-144	140-155	149-168
6 ft. 0 in.	138-144	144-159	153-173

*With shoes—2-in. heels.

For girls 18-25, subtract 1 pound for each year under 25.

height*	small frame	medium frame	large frame
5 ft. 2 in.	112-120	118-129	126-141
5 ft. 3 in.	115-123	121-133	129-144
5 ft. 4 in.	118-126	124-136	132-148
5 ft. 5 in.	121-129	127-139	135-152
5 ft. 6 in.	124-133	130-143	138-156
5 ft. 7 in.	128-137	134-147	142-161
5 ft. 8 in.	132-141	138-152	147-166
5 ft. 9 in.	136-145	142-156	151-170
5 ft. 10 in.	140-150	146-160	155-174
5 ft. 11 in.	144-154	150-165	159-179
6 ft. 0 in.	148-158	154-170	164-184
6 ft. 1 in.	152-162	158-175	168-189
6 ft. 2 in.	156-167	162-180	173-194
6 ft. 3 in.	160-171	167-185	178-199
6 ft. 4 in.	164-175	172-190	182-204

*With shoes—1-in. heels.

Prepared by the Metropolitan Life Insurance Co. from data of the Build and Blood Pressure Study, 1959, Society of Actuaries.